LUNCH AND DINNER

FROM THE

VERY HUNGRY GREEK

First published in Great Britain in 2023 by Yellow Kite
An imprint of Hodder & Stoughton
An Hachette UK company

3

A CIP catalogue record for this title is available from the British Library

Hardback ISBN 978 1 399 71928 5
eBook ISBN 978 1 399 71929 2

Executive Publisher: Liz Gough
Project Editor: Olivia Nightingall
Copyeditor: Vicky Orchard
Design: Hart Studio
Brand Design: hollystead.com
Photography: Ellis Parrinder
Food Stylist: Kate Wesson
Props Stylist: Max Robinson
Senior Production Controller: Matt Everett

Colour origination by Alta Image London
Printed and bound in Italy by Printer Trento S.r.l

Hodder & Stoughton policy is to use papers that are natural, renewable and recyclable products and made from wood grown in sustainable forests. The logging and manufacturing processes are expected to conform to the environmental regulations of the country of origin.

Yellow Kite
Hodder & Stoughton Ltd
Carmelite House
50 Victoria Embankment
London
EC4Y 0DZ

yellowkitebooks.co.uk
www.hodder.co.uk

LUNCH AND DINNER

FROM THE

VERY HUNGRY GREEK

CHRISTINA KYNIGOS

100 QUICK HEALTHY RECIPES UNDER 500 CALORIES

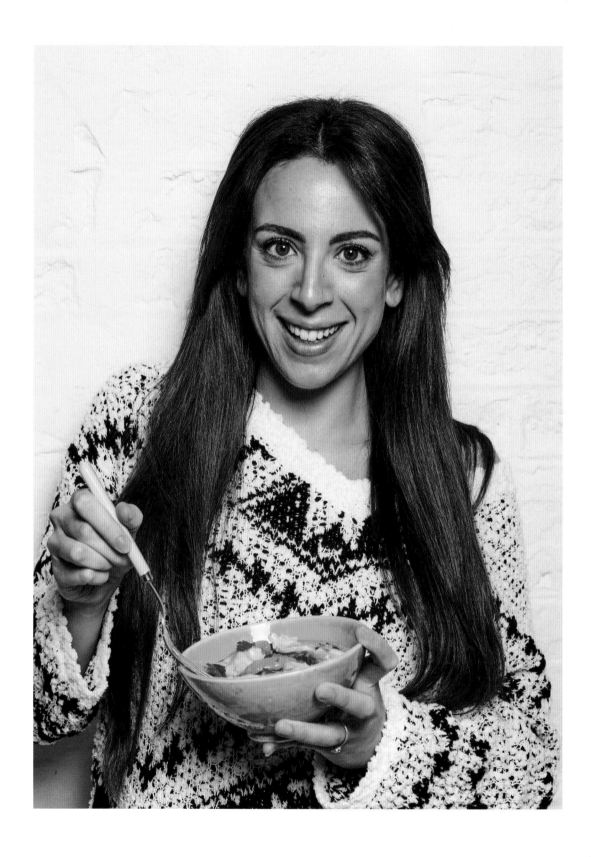

CONTENTS

INTRODUCTION

Hi, I'm Christina (aka the Very Hungry Greek).

Food has always been a massive part of my life, especially growing up in a Greek-Cypriot household. Big portions were normal and having seconds (sometimes thirds) wasn't frowned upon but admired. So, when I noticed that I was piling on the pounds without thinking about my waistline, I knew I had to do something about it.

But how could I stop eating all my favourite foods? Why should I have to? So, I came up with a solution and started creating my own recipes that tasted like all of my favourite foods and takeaways, using swaps to keep the calories down but keeping tons of flavour. I made sure my dishes were low-calorie and healthy, yet mouth-watering and indulgent. Think cheese-pulls, carbs and a good drizzle of your favourite sauce.

At first, I started creating recipes for my own use, but I was being asked left, right and centre to share the recipes on Instagram. When that took off in 2020 and led to the creation of my first book, I wanted to see where else I could share my recipes and help people cook healthily without any restrictions, so I decided to start a TikTok account in 2021. It was a hit, and I couldn't believe the response I was getting, but, looking after more social media platforms, my day job was getting too stressful and – quite honestly – unbearable. I wanted to dedicate all my time to cooking and sharing my recipes with the world and knew this was my calling.

So, I took the plunge, quit my 9 to 5 in 2022, and I'm now a full-time recipe developer and content creator, which has led to this second cookbook, working with some fantastic brands and waking up in the morning with a massive smile on my face.

I hope you love my recipes as much as I've loved creating them! There are no restrictions here and never will be. Healthy food will never be boring again!

Love,

Christina

ABOUT THE BOOK

THE CHAPTERS

I wanted this book to cover the food you will really eat. All the carbs, all the flavour, less of the boring stuff. My recipes aren't like the typical ones you find in most healthy cookbooks, the ones that you flick through and don't ever cook. My recipes will have you cooking your way, hopefully, through the entire book. You'll notice that I haven't included any breakfasts, snacks or desserts here. That's because I did a poll on my social media and found that you all wanted more lunch and dinner inspiration and less of the other stuff. So, I made this book especially for you.

5-INGREDIENT MEALS

Perfect for when you don't want the hassle of a long list of ingredients but still fancy something super tasty. This chapter was inspired by a series I created for my social media platforms that blew up, so I had to put it in the book! My Cheesy Taco Orzo recipe (see page 15) was the biggest hit with over 1 million views. Please note that storecupboard herbs, spices and oils are not included in the 5 'main ingredients' as hopefully you will already have at least some of these to hand. Optional suggestions are also not included as these are extras which you can add if you have them.

STREET FOOD

Whenever I go to a street food market, I want to try everything in sight. From foods I'm familiar with to those completely out of the ordinary, that's what makes street food so diverse and appealing. I've got something for everyone in this chapter and I've loaded it with plenty of lunch-style recipes like wraps, toasties and quick Mexican food to rustle up when you're in a hurry.

PASTA HEAVEN

I couldn't choose just one or two pasta recipes, so I had to dedicate a whole chapter to this heavenly carb. Remember: carbs are fuel! There's no reason to think that you can't eat them when you're eating healthily. If you love lasagne but fancy something a bit different, you've got to try the Lasagne Pockets (see page 84) while the Tuscan Pasta recipe (see page 67) is my favourite pasta dish I've ever made.

ONE-POT WONDERS

Who doesn't love a one-pot wonder? In my eyes, less washing up is like the holy grail after a long day at work. If you love Thai food, this chapter has two amazingly fragrant recipes – Thai green and red curry – to get your teeth stuck into (see page 93). If you're a meatball fan and a little obsessed like me, I've also included two meatball dishes here for you to try (see pages 99 and 106).

MEAL PREP WARRIORS

Do you meal prep on the weekend for the week ahead? If your answer is yes, this chapter will be your new best friend. These freezeable, mouth-watering recipes will not only excite you but will help you to stick to your nutritional goals. The Sloppy Joe Nachos (see page 128) are so addictive that you'll want to stick your face straight into them, the Southern Not-so-Fried Chicken and Slaw (see page 139) tastes like you're eating something super naughty, and the Mexican Chicken Tortilla Soup with crushed tortillas (see page 123) is one of the most filling, flavourful soups that I've ever made . . . YUM.

FAKEAWAYS

Fakeaways are just magical, and I make sure mine taste as identical as possible to a takeaway but with half the calories and all the indulgence. The Kebab Fakeaway Box (see page 161) and Crispy Chicken Rice Box (see page 148) both have it all and are great for you and the family to get stuck into, but the Cheeseburger Calzone (see page 166) will leave you wondering how on earth it's low-calorie with its mouth-watering dough and indulgent filling.

CROWD-PLEASERS

If you've got guests coming round or fancy impressing your partner or housemates, give these crowd-pleasers a go and you'll soon be turning to them as weekly staples. Choosing a favourite from this chapter is a toughie, but the dishes I make time and time again have got to be the Pork Katsu Curry (see page 187 – I like to use chicken sometimes too) and the Creamy Chicken, Leek and Mushroom Filo Pie (see page 190). If you're looking for your Greek fix, the Moussaka (see page 174) is a real hit and if you love burgers, the Garlic Bread Peri-Peri Chicken Burger (see page 178) will become the new love of your life.

BUDGET BANGERS

For anyone on a budget or if you don't want to pay an arm and a leg for a scrummy meal, this chapter is perfect. Each dish comes to less than £1.50 a serving (subject to change with inflation over time!) but that depends on where you shop. I'm a massive fan of Aldi and think their produce is great, which always keeps the cost of a weekly shop down if you want to save some pennies. I'm a huge fan of the Smoky Sausage Foil Parcels (see page 199) as they're so easy to throw together and you can eat them out of the parcels, which even saves on washing up!

THE RECIPES

CALORIE COUNT

I use a calorie counter app called Calorie Counter by Nutracheck to track all the calories and macros in these recipes. I think it's fab, is a lot more user-friendly than other apps I've tried in the past and has a great user interface. You do have to pay a couple of quid a month for it but it's not blowing the bank and totally worth it compared to the free apps.

All ingredients listed in the recipes, excluding those marked as optional, are included in the calorie count. Side suggestions to serve with the recipes, for example carbs and veg, are not included in the calories as they are subject to what you pick and the quantity you choose. It's also worth bearing in mind that some calories count more than others – take 100g broccoli vs 100g chips. The broccoli would come to 34 calories, yet the chips, for the same amount, gives you 165 calories. Broccoli is high in water and fibre, which create bulk without contributing significant calories, whereas potatoes are full of starch, are incredibly filling and are higher in calories. It's important to think about this when eating healthily but still want to include all of your favourite food groups to enjoy a balanced diet.

MACROS

For some, macros (fat, protein and carbohydrates) are important to measure. For example, if you're trying to reach certain fitness goals like building muscle and losing fat, counting macros is essential as you need to consume specific amounts of macronutrients in order to boost performance and gain lean body mass. As with the calorie counts, I also use the Calorie Counter by Nutracheck app to calculate the macros for each recipe, so I've done the hard work for you.

DIETARY REQUIREMENTS

Look out for the information at the start of each recipe, which states the dietary information for that recipe. Remember to always check the packaging if you have a certain dietary requirement; for example, when using vegetable stock, do double check it's gluten-free and always check the swaps section, which features simple suggestions for making recipes suitable for free-from diets – for example switching soy sauce for tamari to make a dish gluten-free. I've also included handy icons to show where meals are freezer-friendly and if they can be cooked in an air fryer. Air fryers are more energy-efficient than using your oven; you don't need to preheat them, and you can cook food quicker. Win-win! For a freezer-friendly recipe, make sure you leave the food to cool before transferring it to an airtight container. For any recipes that are marked as freezer-friendly and have a salad or sauce as a side, remove from the container before heating and/or don't freeze those elements.

VE	Vegan	NF	Nut-free
V	Vegetarian	❄	Freezer-friendly
GF	Gluten-free		Air fryer cooking option
DF	Dairy-free		

LOOK OUT FOR THESE IN THE RECIPES:

Tips: When creating these recipes, I thought of some tips to share with you that might come in handy when you make these recipes at home.

Swaps: If you don't eat a certain type of meat or have a dietary requirement, I've highlighted swaps for you to show what can be easily changed.

Optionals: These suggestions could take your recipes to the next level if you fancy jazzing them up a bit! All the recipes will still taste fab without them, but the optional ingredients are basically the cherry on the cake, if they float your boat, of course.

Side suggestions: Not all the recipes need to be served with something else, for example, if the recipe already has 2 out of your 5-a-day, or has a carb included in the main ingredients. But for the recipes that need that extra fibre and carbs to turn them into a full meal, make sure you have a look at the side suggestions. They are normally a carb like rice or potatoes and some veg.

Oven temperatures: I use a fan oven, but if you've got a conventional oven at home, increase the temperature by 20°C for each recipe. You'll find a handy conversion chart for oven temperatures, as well as for metric to imperial weights, on page 224.

KEY INGREDIENTS

Lean protein – If you're anything like me, crispy bacon fat or chicken skin is IMPOSSIBLE to resist. So, cut out the temptation and buy lean meat to save on a load of calories. Try and choose the 5% lean beef mince and make sure to remove all fat from chicken, pork, lamb, beef and bacon. Chicken thighs mentioned in recipes are skinless and boneless.

Low-fat dairy – Fat-free Greek yogurt, reduced-fat soft cheese, low-fat butter and semi-skimmed milk are your go-to buys for low-fat dairy products.

Bread – Tortilla wraps and gluten-free rolls are wonderfully low in calories, while anything wholemeal, which fills you up for longer, features a lot in this book. Panko breadcrumbs are something I use regularly to make an amazing crispy coating, but you can blitz toasted gluten-free or wholemeal bread to make your own too.

Pasta, rice, beans and pulses – Yes . . . all the carbs! They're handy to have in the cupboard, quick to rustle up a meal with and great for bulking up curries, stews and soups. Pasta is also amazingly versatile.

Low-calorie cooking spray – Essential for cutting down the calories when frying food. The oil sprays are great, get food super crispy and you know exactly what's in them.

Stock pots – Swap your standard stock cube for a stock pot; they're bursting with flavour and come in a variety of different flavours like chicken, beef and veg. I promise you'll never go back to stock cubes again!

Herbs and spices – I'm all about food that packs a flavour punch, and I don't hold back on dried seasonings. My motto is: don't be shy and experiment! Sometimes I want convenience and pre-mixed seasonings are brilliant for that, so you'll find taco seasoning, chicken seasoning and tandoori spices featured in many of my recipes.

Aromatics – Fresh herbs, ginger, garlic, red chilli and citrus fruits like lemons and limes are brilliant for adding a zing of flavour and are used in lots of my recipes.

5-INGREDIENT MEALS

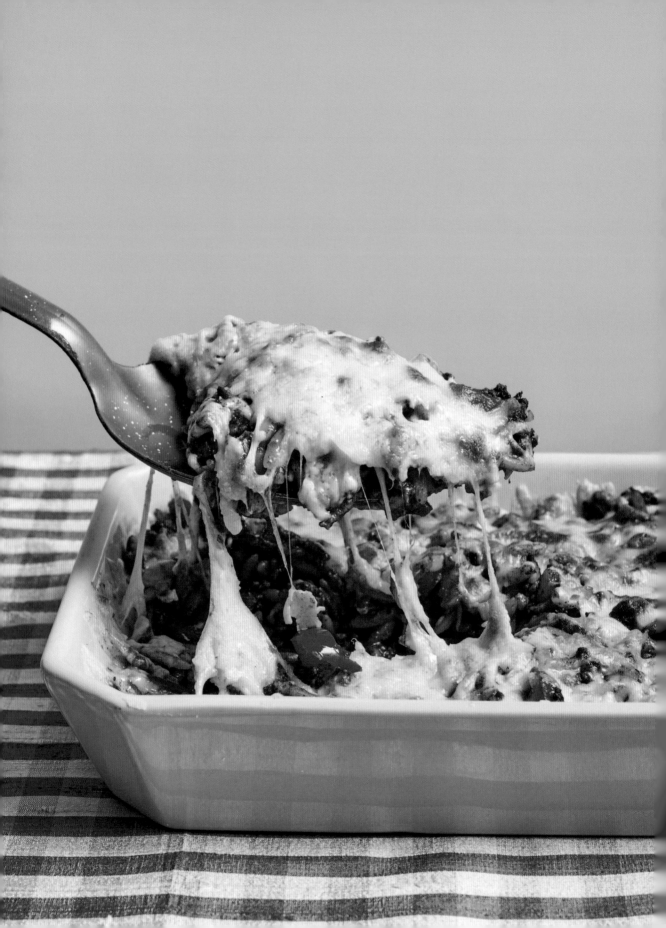

CHEESY TACO ORZO

SERVES: 2 | **PREP:** 2 MINS | **COOK:** 10–12 MINS | NF

If you haven't tried orzo, it's a tiny pasta in the shape of a large rice grain. I've added cheesy beef mince flavoured with taco seasoning to it, along with red peppers to get your veg in.

Main ingredients
100g orzo

250g lean beef mince

1 heaped tbsp
tomato purée

1 red pepper,
finely diced

50g reduced-fat
Cheddar, grated

Herbs, spices and oils
Low-calorie
cooking spray

20g taco seasoning
sachet

Salt and pepper

Swap: Make this dish veggie by using veggie mince.

Cook the orzo in boiling salted water according to the packet instructions. Drain, reserving a ladle of pasta water, and set aside.

Meanwhile, spray a frying pan with low-calorie cooking spray and fry the beef mince for 4–5 minutes. Sprinkle over the taco seasoning, then add the tomato purée and the ladle of pasta water. Add the finely diced pepper and cook for a further 3–4 minutes. Mix everything together, then season with a pinch of salt and pepper.

Stir in most of the Cheddar and, once the cheese has melted, transfer to an ovenproof dish, top with the remaining Cheddar and place under a hot grill until the cheese has melted.

KCAL	CARBS	PROTEIN	FAT	❄
433	45g	44g	8g	

CHICKEN TIKKA FLATBREAD

SERVES: 2 | **PREP**: 2 MINS (+15 MINS MARINATING) | **COOK**: 6–8 MINS | NF

The quickest chicken tikka you will ever make, paired with homemade minted yogurt smothered on a flatbread. Don't forget a spoonful of mango chutney!

Main ingredients

4 heaped tbsp 0% fat Greek yogurt

2 chicken breasts, sliced

2 flatbreads

2 handfuls of iceberg lettuce, sliced

Sliced red onion

Sliced cucumber (optional)

Mango chutney, to serve (optional)

Herbs, spices and oils

4–5 mint leaves, finely chopped

4 tsp tikka curry paste

Low-calorie cooking spray

In a small bowl, mix the mint and 3 heaped tablespoons of the yogurt together and place in the fridge. In a bowl, mix the tikka paste and 1 tablespoon of yogurt together, then marinade the chicken in this mixture for at least 15 minutes.

Spray a pan with low-calorie cooking spray and fry the chicken slices for 6–7 minutes or until cooked. Dice the chicken into small pieces.

Lightly toast the flatbreads, then spread the minty yogurt mixture over each one. Top with the lettuce, red onion and diced chicken and serve.

Optional: Add more salad, such as cucumber, then a drizzle of mango chutney on top of the chicken.

Air fryer method: Air-fry the chicken at 200°C for 5 minutes before flipping, spraying with a little more low-calorie cooking spray and air-frying for another 5 minutes, or until cooked.

KCAL	CARBS	PROTEIN	FAT	
424	39g	53g	6g	

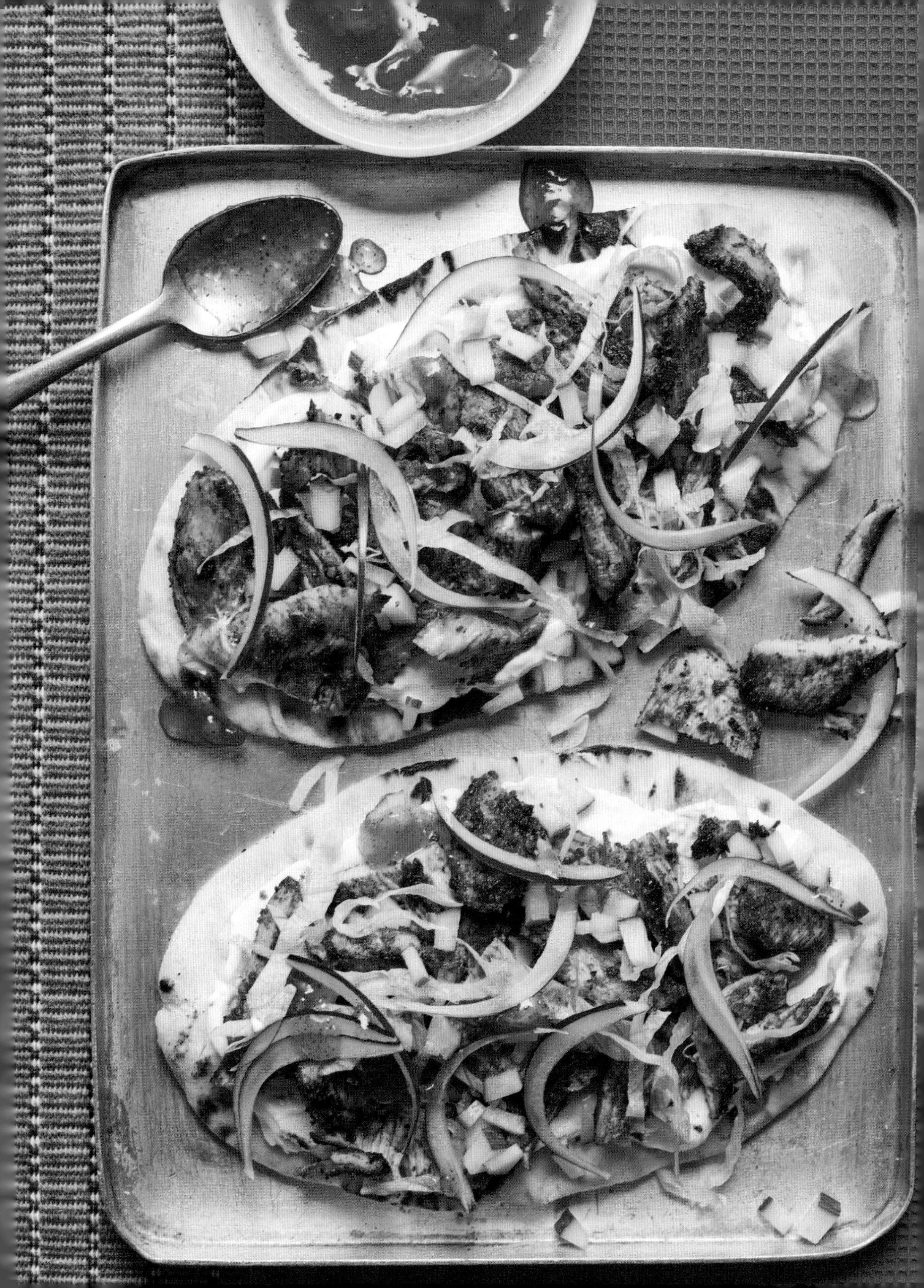

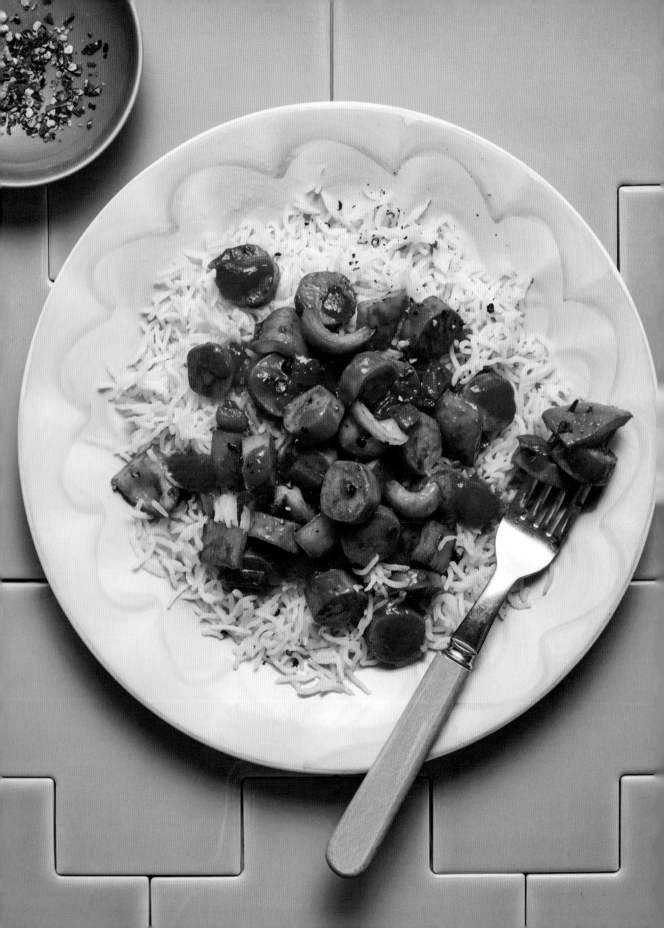

CHILLI SAUSAGES

SERVES: 3 | PREP: 2 MINS | COOK: 6–8 MINS | DF + NF

If you like a bit of a kick to your meals and love frankfurter sausages, then look no further. The sausages are spiced with chilli flakes and mixed with a tangy tomato sauce.

Main ingredients
1 red onion, diced

1 green pepper, diced

10 frankfurter sausages, sliced

2 tbsp soy sauce

3 tbsp reduced-sugar tomato ketchup

Herbs, spices and oils
Low-calorie cooking spray

½ tsp garlic granules

1 tsp chilli powder of your choice

1–2 tsp chilli flakes

Side suggestion
Basmati rice

Swaps: Swap the frankfurters for reduced-fat pork or chicken sausages and use tamari instead of soy sauce to make this gluten-free!

Spray a frying pan with low-calorie cooking spray and fry the onion and green pepper for 2–3 minutes to soften. (Don't like your veg with a bite? Add a dash of water to soften it further.)

Mix in the frankfurter sausages and garlic granules, then fry for a further 3–4 minutes. Add the remaining ingredients and fry for a further minute, making sure the sauce coats everything nicely.

KCAL	CARBS	PROTEIN	FAT	
380	11g	17g	30g	

FISH FINGER PIE

SERVES: 4 | **PREP:** 5 MINS | **COOK:** 25 MINS | NF

The simplest fish pie and instead of using fish pieces, I've changed it up by using shop-bought breaded fish fingers as anything breaded takes a dish to the next level.

Main ingredients

2 potatoes, peeled and cubed

135ml semi-skimmed milk

200g frozen peas, defrosted

12 fish fingers, cooked

125g reduced-fat Cheddar, grated

Herbs, spices and oils

A knob of butter (optional)

Salt and pepper

Boil the cubed potatoes in salted water for 20 minutes or until tender. Drain, pour in the milk, add a pinch of salt and pepper and mash until smooth. Mix in the peas.

Place the fish fingers at the bottom of a large ovenproof dish, add the mash on top, then the grated cheese. Place under a hot grill for a couple of minutes until the cheese is golden.

Optional: Mix a knob of butter into the mash for extra creaminess and indulgence.

KCAL	CARBS	PROTEIN	FAT	
370	42g	30g	10g	

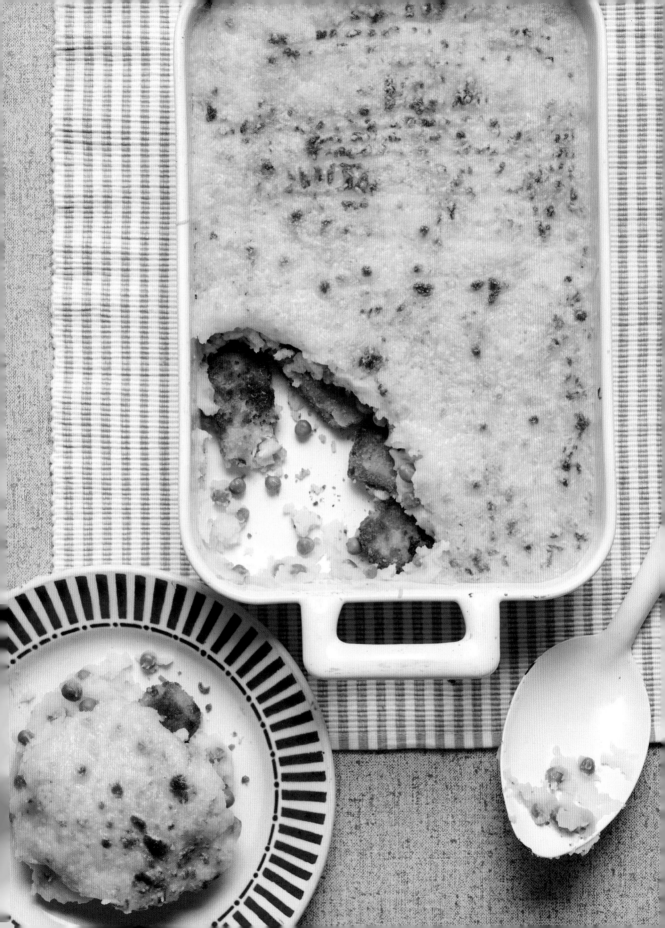

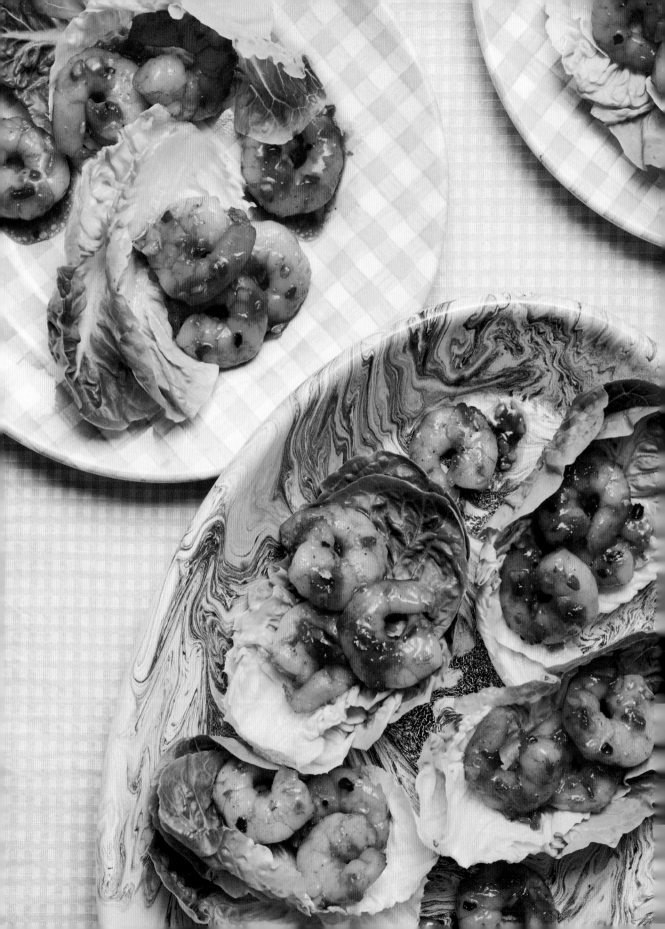

SWEET CHILLI PRAWN LETTUCE CUPS

SERVES: 2 | **PREP**: 2 MINS | **COOK**: 4 MINS | DF + NF

Bite-sized lettuce cups of pure bliss. These king prawns are coated in a sticky, sweet chilli glaze and make a great appetiser or protein-fuelled snack.

Main ingredients

360g king prawns, peeled and deveined

2 garlic cloves, minced

8 little gem lettuce leaves

Herbs, spices and oils

60g reduced-sugar sweet chilli sauce

2 tsp soy sauce

Low-calorie cooking spray

Swap: To make this gluten-free, swap the soy sauce for tamari.

Mix 40g of the sweet chilli sauce and the soy sauce together and set aside.

Spray a frying pan with low-calorie cooking spray and fry the king prawns on a low–medium heat for 2 minutes on each side, along with the garlic. For the last 30 seconds, crank up the heat and pour in the sauce, making sure the prawns are well coated.

Place the prawns in the lettuce leaves, then drizzle over the remaining sweet chilli sauce and enjoy!

KCAL	CARBS	PROTEIN	FAT
188	12g	30g	2g

HONEY CHILLI HALLOUMI AND CHORIZO PITTA

SERVES: 2 | **PREP:** 2 MINS | **COOK:** 6–8 MINS | NF

Being slightly biased because I'm Greek-Cypriot, halloumi is an ingredient I can eat daily. Grilled halloumi is wonderful as is, but here I've fried it with honey and chilli for a warming but sweet flavour and added smoky chorizo in a salad-filled pitta.

Main ingredients

1 tbsp honey
Squeeze of lemon juice
30g chorizo, sliced
90g light halloumi, sliced
2 pittas, toasted
2 handfuls of mixed salad or rocket (optional)
8 cherry tomatoes, sliced (optional)

Herbs, spices and oils

Pinch of chilli flakes

In a small bowl, mix together the honey, chilli flakes and lemon juice, then set aside.

In a frying pan, fry the sliced chorizo on a low–medium heat for 2–3 minutes to release the oils, then set aside. In the same pan, fry the halloumi for a few minutes until golden, then pour over the honey sauce.

Fry for a further minute or two on a medium heat to coat the halloumi. Grab a toasted pitta, cut into a pocket and add the rocket and cherry tomatoes (if using), along with the halloumi and chorizo.

Air fryer method: Coat the halloumi slices in the honey, chilli and lemon juice, then air-fry with the chorizo at 200°C for 5 minutes.

KCAL	CARBS	PROTEIN	FAT
381	39g	22g	15g

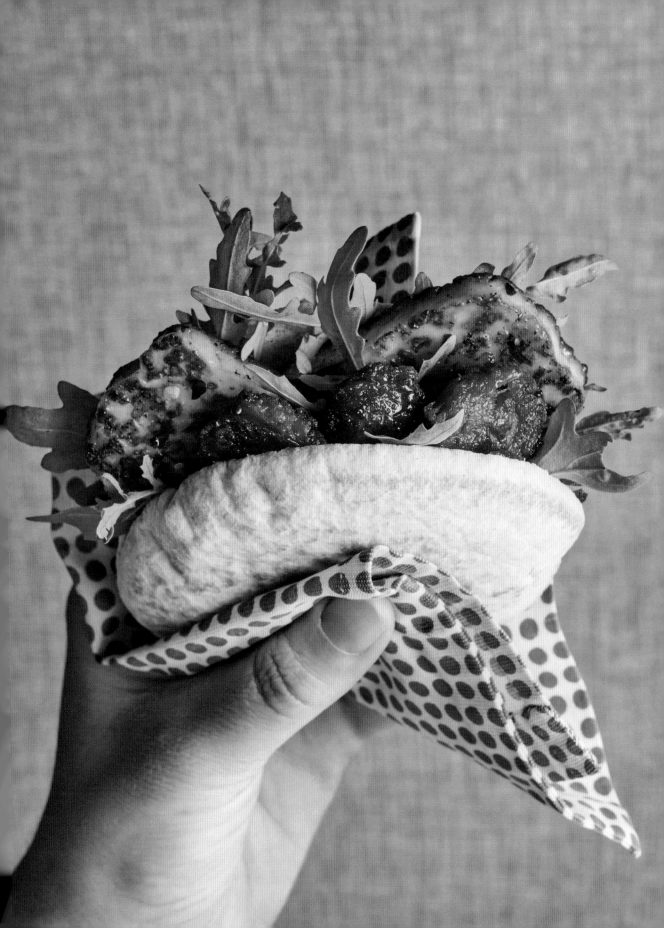

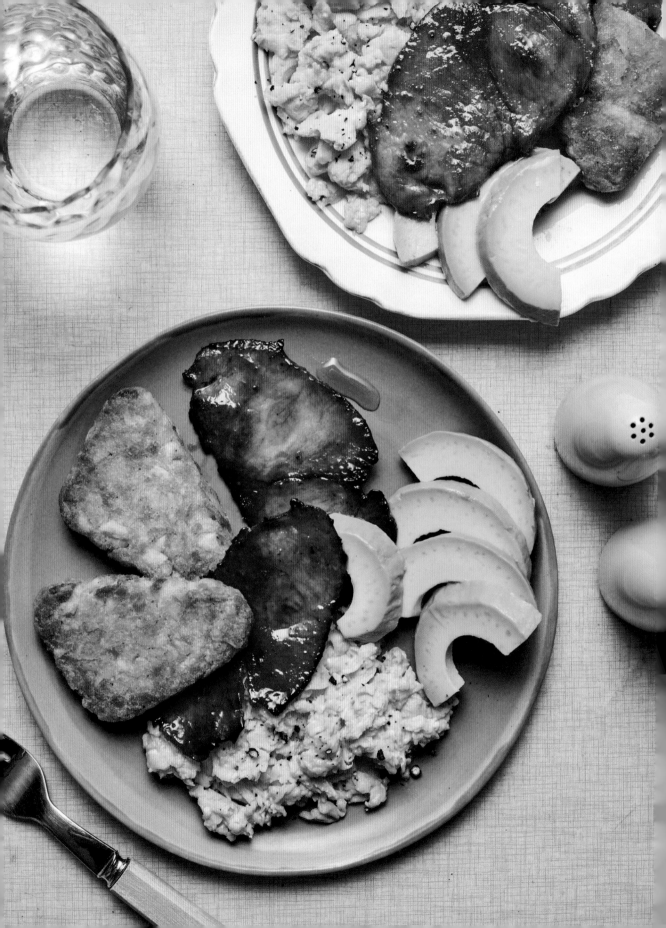

MAPLE BACON AND HASH BROWN BRUNCH PLATE

SERVES: 2 | **PREP:** 5 MINS | **COOK:** 6–8 MINS | GF + DF + NF

Bacon glazed with maple syrup paired with scrambled eggs and golden hash browns, topped with creamy sliced avocado, this is a breakfast (or brunch) of champions.

Main ingredients

4 smoked bacon medallions
2 tsp maple syrup
4 eggs
4 hash browns, cooked
½ avocado, sliced

Herbs, spices and oils

Low-calorie cooking spray
Salt and pepper

Swap: If you don't fancy bacon, swap it for chorizo instead.

Fry the bacon in low-calorie cooking spray for a couple of minutes until cooked. Crank up the heat, then add the maple syrup. Coat the bacon well and fry for a further minute, then remove from the pan.

Scramble the eggs in a pan with low-calorie cooking spray for a couple of minutes until cooked. Season with salt and pepper.

Plate up the hash browns, scrambled eggs, bacon and sliced avocado and enjoy.

KCAL	CARBS	PROTEIN	FAT
484	24g	27g	30g

CRISPY PANCETTA, PEA AND POTATO SKILLET

SERVES: 2 | **PREP:** 2 MINS | **COOK:** 10–12 MINS | GF + NF

The contrast of salty pancetta with the freshness of the peas takes this dish to another level, all teamed up with crushed new potatoes for a carb filling factor.

Main ingredients
90g pancetta, diced
560g tinned new
   potatoes
150g peas, cooked
40g reduced-fat
   Cheddar

**Herbs, spices
and oils**
Salt and pepper
1 tsp paprika

**Swaps: You can use
bacon medallions to
save on the calories
and cooked new
potatoes instead
of tinned ones.**

Fry the pancetta in a frying pan on a medium–high heat for 3–4 minutes until crispy then remove and set aside, leaving any fat in the pan. Place the new potatoes in the same pan and crush with the back of a mug, pressing down gently.

Season with pepper and half the paprika, then without moving the potatoes, fry on a high heat for 2 minutes. Flip, season again using the remaining paprika, salt and pepper and fry for a further 2 minutes. Scatter over the peas, then add the pancetta and cheese.

Either place a lid over the pan to melt the cheese or place the pan under a hot grill for a few minutes.

Air fryer method: Place the crushed potatoes and pancetta in a foil parcel in the air fryer and spray with plenty of low-calorie cooking spray, then season with salt and pepper. Air-fry at 200°C for 10–15 minutes, flipping halfway. Scatter over the peas and the cheese, then place back in the air fryer and cook for a further few minutes.

KCAL	CARBS	PROTEIN	FAT		
495	51g	23g	22g		

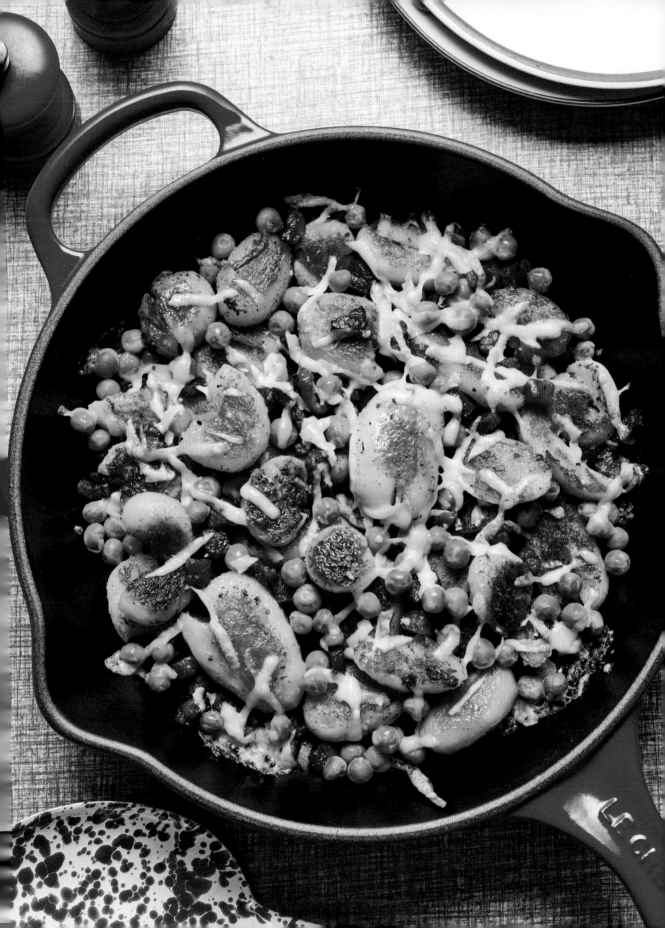

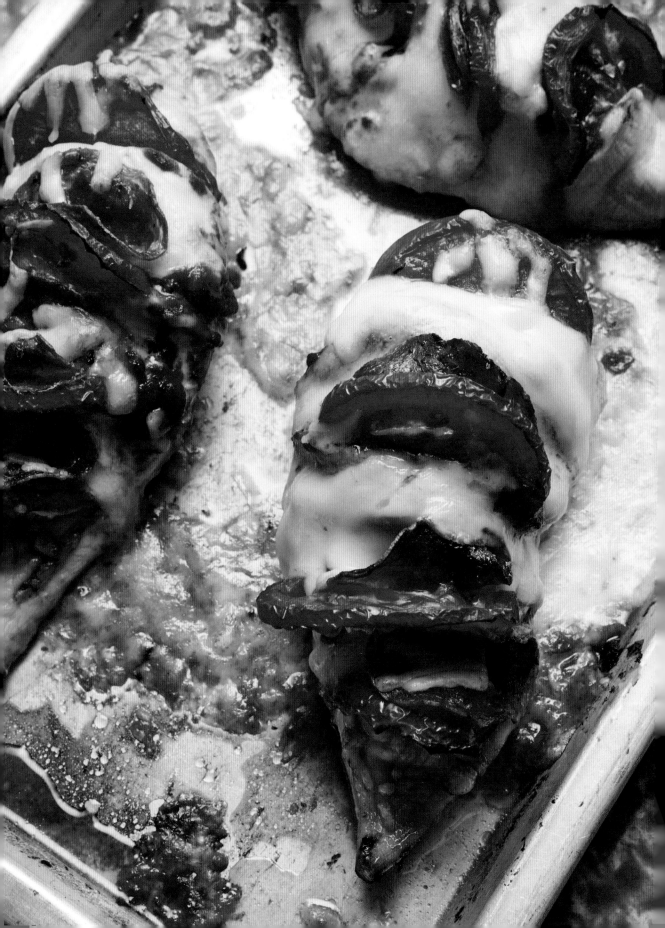

HASSELBACK PEPPERONI PIZZA CHICKEN

SERVES: 4 | PREP: 5 MINS | COOK: 20 MINS | GF + NF

All the delicious flavours of a pepperoni pizza to spice up plain old chicken breasts. A one-pot wonder and a fuss-free meal you can serve with just about anything.

Main ingredients
4 chicken breasts
4 tbsp tomato purée
4 tomatoes, sliced
200g reduced-fat mozzarella, sliced
16 pepperoni slices
A handful of grated Cheddar (optional)

Herbs, spices and oils
2 tsp dried oregano
Salt and pepper

Side suggestions
Any types of carbs like mash or chips, or a simple side salad

Swap: Sliced mushrooms or peppers also work in place of the tomatoes.

Preheat the oven to 190°C.

Make 4 deep cuts in each chicken breast, nearly going to the bottom but not all the way through, then season well with salt and pepper.

In a small bowl, mix together the tomato purée, oregano and 4–5 tablespoons of water to loosen the mixture. Spread this mixture into each of the cuts.

Add a slice of tomato to each of the cuts, along with a slice of mozzarella, pepperoni, a sprinkle of the Cheddar (if using), then place on a lined baking tray.

Bake in the oven for 20 minutes or until cooked.

Air fryer method: Air-fry the stuffed chicken at 190°C for 20 minutes.

KCAL	CARBS	PROTEIN	FAT		
385	7g	54g	16g	❄️	

PONZU CHICKEN WITH CRISPY SMASHED POTATOES

SERVES: 4 | **PREP**: 2 MINS (+30 MINS MARINATING) | **COOK**: 12–15 MINS | DF + NF

Ponzu is a classic Japanese condiment and has a tangy, citrus flavour. Not only does this recipe taste great, but it looks pretty cool with the criss-cross sliced chicken breasts.

Main ingredients

4 tbsp soy sauce

2 tbsp honey

Juice of ½ lemon

4 chicken breasts

700g new potatoes, cooked

Herbs, spices and oils

3–4 garlic cloves, minced

2 tsp sesame oil

Low-calorie cooking spray

Side suggestions

Tenderstem broccoli

Lemon wedges

Swap: Use tamari instead of soy sauce to make this gluten-free.

Preheat the oven to 200°C.

Mix all the ingredients, except the chicken, new potatoes and low-calorie cooking spray, together to make the marinade and set aside.

Score one side of the chicken breasts in a criss-cross pattern and place in the marinade, scored side down, making sure they are all well coated. Marinade for at least 30 minutes but overnight is best for an intense flavour.

Spray a frying pan with low-calorie cooking spray and fry the chicken breasts for 5–6 minutes on each side. If you have any remaining marinade, drizzle this over for the last minute of cooking. Remove the chicken from the pan and leave to rest for at least 4–5 minutes before serving.

At the same time, spray a lined baking tray with low-calorie cooking spray and add the cooked potatoes. Using the back of a mug, lightly push down to smash each potato. Spray with more low-calorie cooking spray and cook at 200°C for 10–15 minutes.

Air fryer method: Air-fry the marinated chicken at 200°C for 15–20 minutes. For the last few minutes, glaze with any remaining marinade. To cook the potatoes, use the back of a mug to lightly push down and smash each potato and place in the air fryer, spray with low-calorie cooking spray and air-fry at 200°C for 8–10 minutes.

KCAL	CARBS	PROTEIN	FAT		
347	31g	34g	4g	❄	

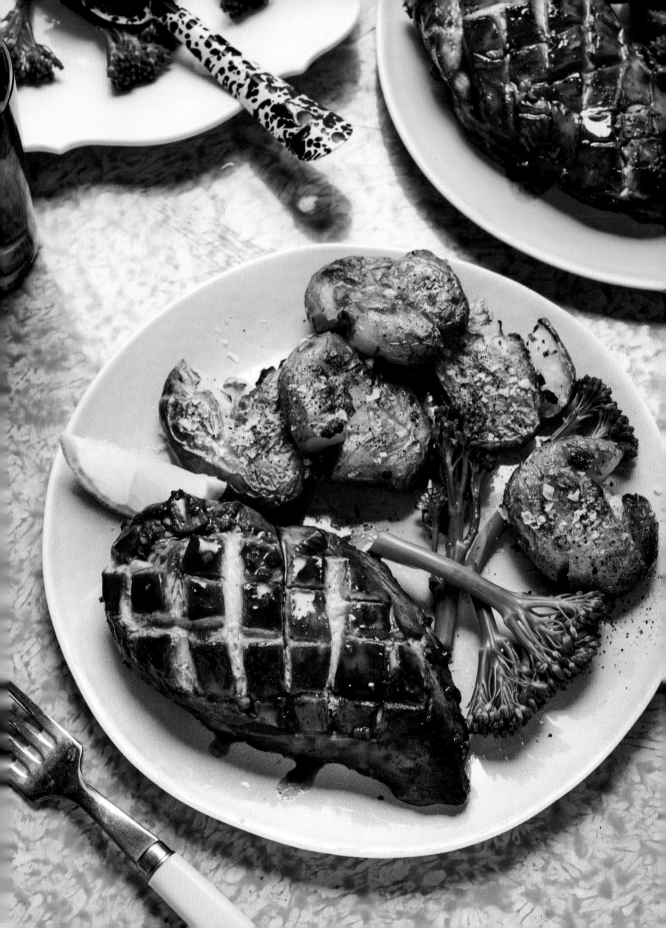

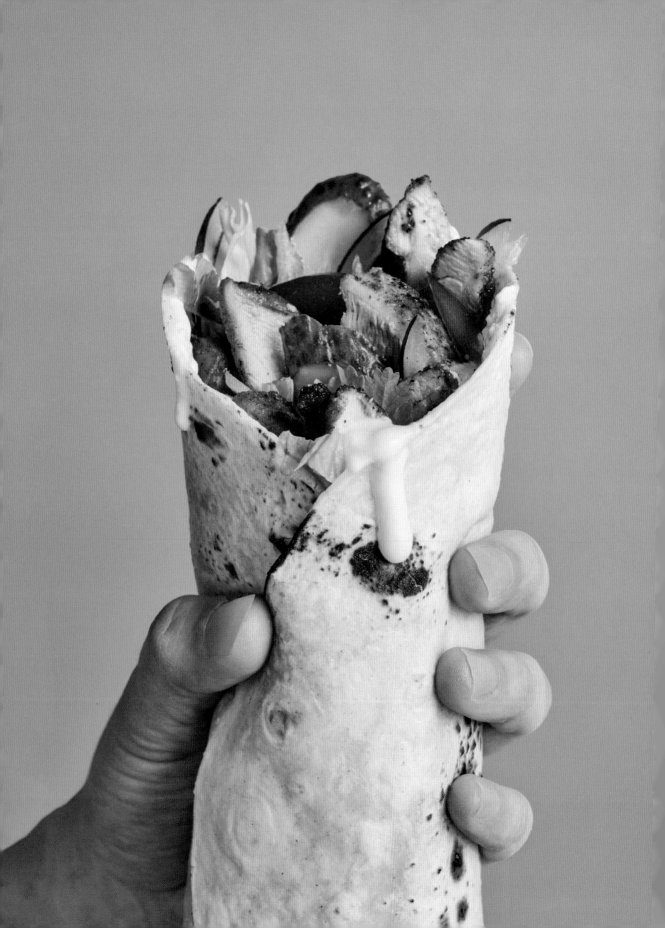

QUICKY SHAWARMA

SERVES: 4 | PREP: 2 MINS (+30 MINS MARINATING) | COOK: 7–8 MINS | NF

Normally layered on a vertical rotisserie or spit where it's slow-roasted, I just had to include a quick shawarma that tastes the same but is made in half the time. You could layer the chicken on a rotisserie stick and place it in the oven, but it works just as well cooked in a pan.

Main ingredients

5 large skinless, boneless chicken thigh fillets

4 tortilla wraps

4 handfuls of iceberg lettuce

4 red onion slices

4 tomatoes, sliced

4 gherkins, sliced (optional)

Fresh coriander, chopped (optional)

Herbs, oils and spices

Low-calorie cooking spray

Marinade

1 tbsp olive oil

1 tsp garlic granules

1 tsp ground cumin

1 tsp ground turmeric

1 tsp paprika

Salt and pepper

Garlic sauce (optional)

4 heaped tbsp 0% fat Greek yogurt

2–3 garlic cloves

Squeeze of lemon juice

Marinate the chicken in all the marinade ingredients for at least 30 minutes or overnight if possible.

Spray a large frying pan with plenty of low-calorie cooking spray and fry the chicken on a medium heat for 6–7 minutes, flipping halfway. Remove from the pan and leave to rest for 6 minutes. (Fry the chicken in batches to not overcrowd the pan if your pan is on the smaller side.) Make sure the chicken is cooked through before dicing it.

If using, blend all the garlic sauce ingredients together and add a dash of water if needed to loosen it.

To assemble the shawarma, spread a layer of your homemade garlic sauce over each wrap, then add the lettuce, red onion, tomatoes and gherkins (if using). Top with the diced chicken and coriander (if using). Wrap and enjoy!

Optional: Add slices of gherkins to the wraps, a sprinkle of fresh coriander and homemade garlic sauce.

Air fryer method: Air-fry the marinated chicken at 200°C for 16–18 minutes, turning halfway.

KCAL	CARBS	PROTEIN	FAT		
386	29g	31g	15g		

HONEY MUSTARD SALMON

SERVES: 4 | PREP: 2 MINS | COOK: 8–10 MINS | GF + NF

Fish is an ingredient I grew up with, but I wanted to shake things up by adding a sauce I would normally use with chicken. If you've ever tried honey mustard dressing and adore it, think of that but warmed up on gorgeous bite-sized pieces of salmon.

Main ingredients

3 tbsp honey

2 tsp wholegrain mustard

4 salmon fillets, skin removed

180g reduced-fat soft cheese

100ml water

Herbs, spices and oils

1 tsp paprika (optional)

2 tsp Italian mixed herbs

Low-calorie cooking spray

Salt and pepper

Side suggestions

Chips, mash or new potatoes

Boiled greens

Swap: Don't fancy salmon? Swap for chicken instead.

In a small bowl, mix together the honey and mustard, and paprika (if using), and set aside.

Slice the salmon fillets into big chunks (I normally slice each fillet 4 times) and season with salt, pepper and the Italian herbs. Spray a frying pan with low-calorie cooking spray and cook the salmon for 4–5 minutes.

Pour over the honey mustard sauce and fry for a minute on a high heat, making sure the salmon pieces are well coated. Mix in the soft cheese and water, then fry for a few minutes or until the sauce has thickened.

Optional: Add 1 teaspoon of paprika for a sweet and peppery flavour pop.

Air fryer method: Air-fry the seasoned salmon at 190°C for 8–10 minutes. Then in a pan, mix together the honey, mustard, cream cheese and water on a medium heat for 1–2 minutes or until it thickens, add the cooked salmon fillets, coat well and serve.

KCAL	CARBS	PROTEIN	FAT		
348	11g	31g	20g	❄	

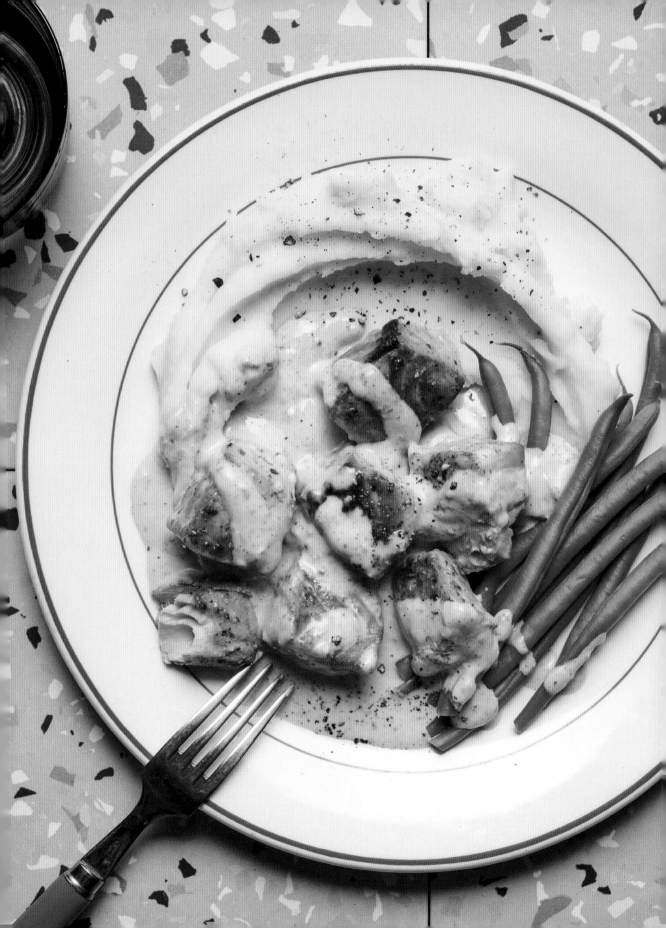

STREET FOOD

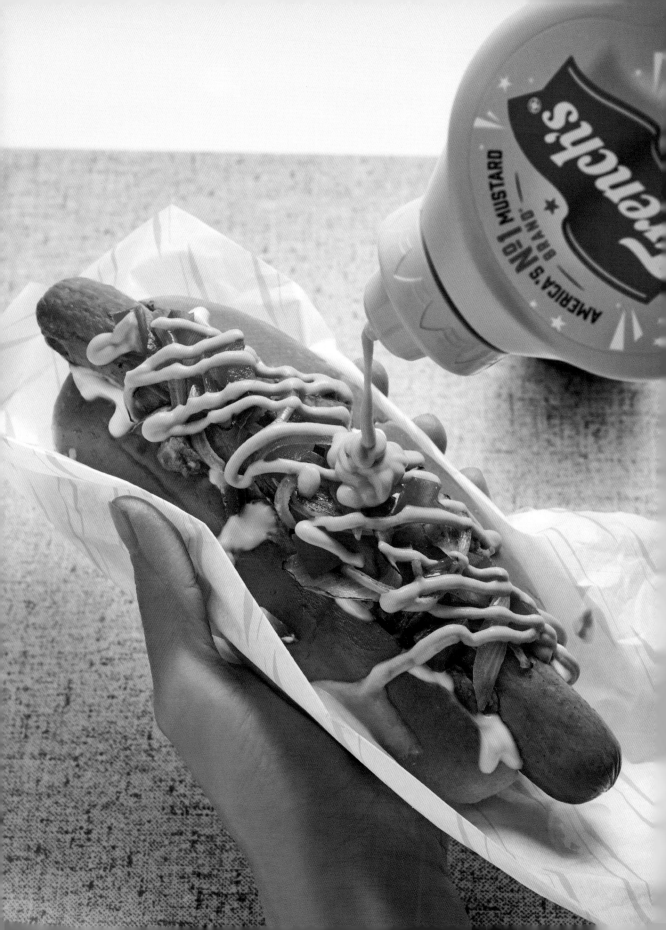

SONORAN HOT DOGS

SERVES: 2 | **PREP**: 2 MINS | **COOK**: 6–8 MINS | DF + NF

This Mexican-style recipe will make sure you never go back to your usual hot dogs ever again. Think streaks of bacon wrapped around a hot dog sausage, with refried beans, jalapeños and topped off with fried mustardy onions. I told you so.

2 hot dog sausages

2 smoked back bacon rashers

Low-calorie cooking spray

½ onion, sliced

1 tsp English mustard

5–6 jalapeño slices, diced

2 hot dog rolls, sliced open

2 tbsp light mayonnaise

4 tbsp refried beans, warmed

1 tomato, finely diced

To serve (optional)
Mustard
Light mayonnaise
Tomato ketchup

Side suggestions
Homemade chips (see page 151)
Slaw

Swap: Streaky bacon works wonderfully with these hot dogs.

Wrap each hot dog sausage with a bacon rasher. Spray a frying pan with low-calorie cooking spray and cook the hot dogs along with the sliced onion for 5–6 minutes, making sure each side of the hot dogs and the onions have browned nicely. Remove the sausages from the pan and set aside.

Add the mustard to the onions, along with the jalapeños, and fry for a further 1–2 minutes.

Assemble the hot dogs by spreading 1 tablespoon of mayonnaise and 2 tablespoons of refried beans on each roll, then add the sausages, onions and jalapeños. Finish off with the diced tomatoes, plus any sauces you fancy.

Optional: Add a drizzle of mustard, more mayonnaise and tomato ketchup on the top.

KCAL	CARBS	PROTEIN	FAT
361	38g	17g	16g

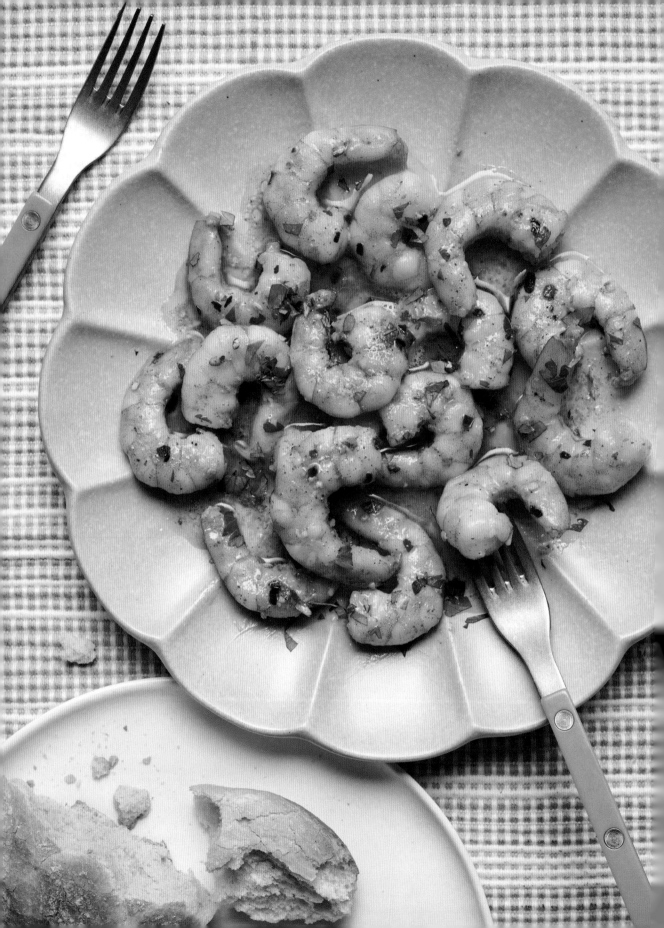

GARLIC BUTTER PRAWNS WITH CRUSTY BREAD

SERVES: 2 | **PREP**: 2 MINS | **COOK**: 7–8 MINS | NF

Just hand me the whole bowl of these and leave me in peace. These are irresistible if you love seafood and the taste of garlic butter. And, to top it off, this recipe calls for you to dip crusty bread into the buttery prawns, just heavenly!

350g raw king prawns, shelled and deveined

2 x 50g bake-at-home rolls, cooked

Garlic butter

2 tbsp low-fat butter

2 tsp olive oil

4 garlic cloves, minced

1 tsp paprika

Pinch of chilli flakes

2 tbsp finely chopped fresh parsley

Heat the butter and oil in a pan, then add all the remaining ingredients, except the rolls, stirring well. Stir-fry the prawns for 4–5 minutes or until cooked through. Serve with the crusty baked rolls.

Air fryer method: Mix all the garlic butter ingredients together, then mix in the king prawns. Air-fry for 5 minutes at 190°C.

KCAL	CARBS	PROTEIN	FAT
388	31g	36g	13g

BOLOGNESE QUESADILLA

SERVES: 4 | **PREP**: 5 MINS | **COOK**: 23–28 MINS | NF

A gorgeous, rich and speedy Bolognese sauce encased in two fried tortilla wraps – who could say no to this invention?

4 tortilla wraps

120g reduced-fat Cheddar

Bolognese

Low-calorie cooking spray

1 red pepper, finely diced

4 mushrooms, finely diced

½ onion, finely diced

250g lean beef mince

½ tsp black pepper

1 tsp mixed herbs

50ml beef stock

500g passata

400g tin chopped tomatoes

Spray a pan with low-calorie cooking spray and fry all the finely diced veg for 3–4 minutes until softened. Add the beef mince and fry for a few minutes until nearly cooked, then mix in the remaining ingredients.

Simmer for about 15 minutes or until the sauce has reduced and all the liquid has evaporated. Remove from the pan and set aside.

Clean the pan, then spray it with low-calorie cooking spray. Fry a tortilla on a medium heat for 1–2 minutes until it starts to crisp up.

Spread half the mixture evenly on top of the tortilla, then add half of the cheese. Immediately place another tortilla over the top and press down gently to enclose. Fry for a further minute, then carefully flip and fry for a further 2 minutes or until browned.

Repeat for the other quesadilla, slice each one into quarters and serve 2 quarters per person.

KCAL	CARBS	PROTEIN	FAT
367	38g	28g	11g

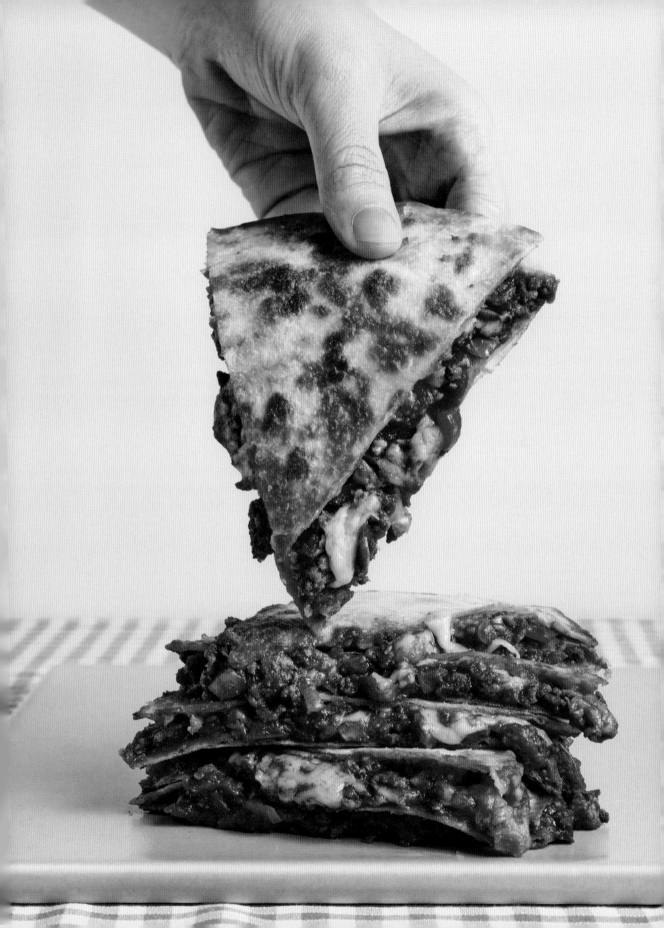

SWEET POTATO AND RED LENTIL DAHL

SERVES: 4 | **PREP**: 5 MINS | **COOK**: 20–25 MINS | VE + GF + DF + NF

I adore lentil curries that are bursting with flavour, and which you can eat bowlfuls of while getting 4 of your 5-a-day in one sitting. Yup – this is the one.

Low-calorie
  cooking spray
½ large onion,
  finely diced
3 garlic cloves, peeled
  and minced
2.5cm piece of fresh
  ginger, minced
1 tbsp garam masala
½ tsp chilli powder
  of your choice
1 tsp ground cumin
¼ tsp ground
  cinnamon
½ tsp ground turmeric
600ml vegetable stock
125g dried red
  split lentils
570g sweet potato,
  peeled and cubed
400g tin chopped
  tomatoes
400ml tin reduced-
  fat coconut milk
Salt and pepper

To serve (optional)
0% fat Greek yogurt
Fresh coriander,
  chopped

Side suggestions
Flatbreads
Naan
Boiled rice

On a low heat, fry the finely diced onion in plenty of low-calorie cooking spray for 2–3 minutes to soften, then add the minced garlic, ginger and spices.

Fry for a few minutes, then add the vegetable stock, lentils and cubed sweet potato. Crank up the heat to high, stir well, then add the chopped tomatoes, coconut milk and a good pinch of salt and pepper. Mix again and cook on a medium–high heat for 15–20 minutes or until the sweet potato has cooked and the stock has reduced. Serve with dollop of 0% fat Greek yogurt and a sprinkle of fresh coriander if you like.

KCAL	CARBS	PROTEIN	FAT
344	57g	12g	9g

CRUNCH WRAP

SERVES: 2 | **PREP:** 2 MINS | **COOK:** 8–9 MINS | NF

As soon as you take that first bite of this wrap you get an amazing crunch from the tortilla chips, combined with tender beef and melted mozzarella. This recipe is perfect to mix and match to your own preferences.

Low-calorie
  cooking spray

150g lean beef mince

4 tsp taco seasoning

3 tbsp tomato salsa

2 tortilla wraps

4 tsp peri-peri
  mayonnaise

50g reduced-fat
  mozzarella, diced

20g chilli tortilla chips

A handful of
  lettuce, sliced

Guacamole (optional)

A few jalapeños
  (optional)

2 mini tortilla wraps

Side suggestion
Side salad

Spray a frying pan with low-calorie cooking spray and fry the beef mince on a medium heat for 3–4 minutes or until cooked. Sprinkle with the taco seasoning, then mix in the salsa, making sure it's evenly combined.

Grab a tortilla wrap, then spread 2 teaspoons of your favourite mayonnaise in the middle of the tortilla (I use peri-peri). Add half the beef mixture, cheese, tortilla chips, lettuce, plus any optional extras, then top with a mini tortilla wrap.

Tightly fold the edges of the tortilla wrap around the mini wrap, then place mini-tortilla-side down in a hot frying pan on a high heat for a few minutes to brown, flipping halfway. (Use low-calorie cooking spray to get it extra crispy.)

Repeat to make the second wrap, slice each wrap in half and enjoy!

Optional: Add a dollop of guacamole and a few jalapeños.

TIP: *Search 'crunch wrap' online as it will help you understand how to fold the wrap.*

KCAL	CARBS	PROTEIN	FAT
472	53g	29g	14g

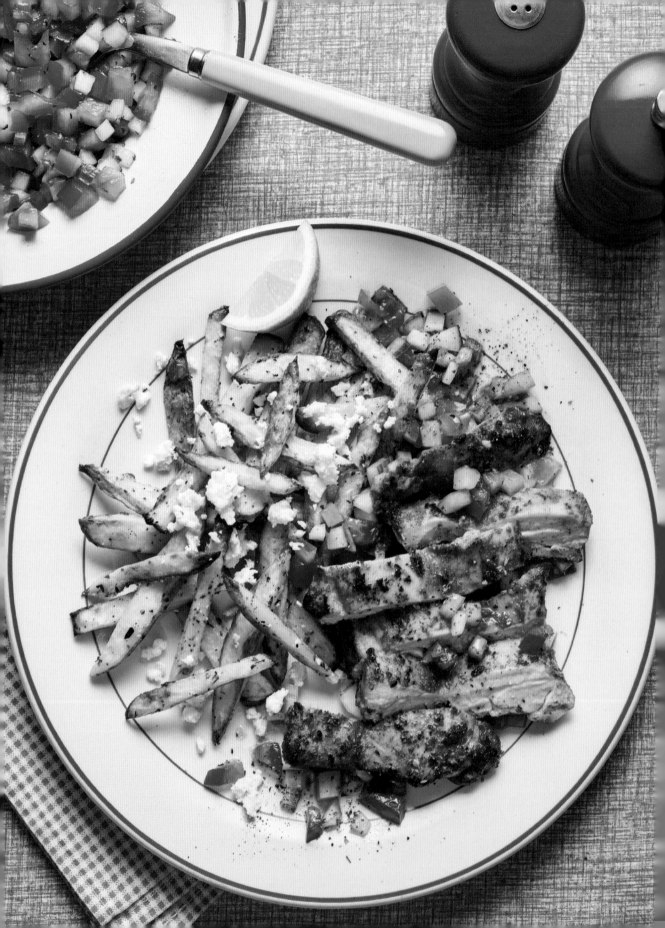

THE ULTIMATE GREEK

SERVES: 2 | **PREP**: 5 MINS (+30 MINS MARINATING) | **COOK**: 15–20 MINS | GF + NF

This is ultimate for a reason. Beautifully marinated gyros-style chicken on top of oregano-seasoned feta fries and a side of yummy Greek salad. This will transport you back to Cyprus or Greece for a celebration of Greek flavours.

Low-calorie cooking spray

Feta chips
2 medium potatoes, sliced into chips
1 tsp dried oregano
30g feta, crumbled
Salt and pepper

Chicken
3 medium skinless, boneless chicken thighs
1 tsp paprika
1 tsp cayenne pepper
½ tsp ground cumin
Squeeze of lemon juice
1 heaped tbsp Greek yogurt
2 garlic cloves, minced

Greek salad
2 tomatoes, finely diced
5cm piece of cucumber, finely diced
2 slices of red onion, finely diced
½ green pepper, finely diced
2 tsp olive oil
Pinch of dried oregano

Marinate the chicken thighs with all the chicken ingredients for at least 30 minutes.

Spray a frying pan with low-calorie cooking spray and fry the chicken thighs on a medium heat for 5–6 minutes on each side. Remove from the pan and leave to rest for 5 minutes before slicing.

Meanwhile, preheat the oven to 180°C.

Place the chips in a large bowl and spray with low-calorie cooking spray. Season with the oregano and a good pinch of salt and pepper. Transfer to a lined baking tray and cook in the oven for 15–20 minutes, turning halfway and spraying with more low-calorie cooking spray. Top with the crumbled feta.

Mix all the salad ingredients together and serve with the sliced chicken and feta chips.

Air fryer method: Place the marinated chicken thighs in the air fryer and spray with low-calorie cooking spray. Air-fry at 200°C for 16 minutes, flipping halfway, then leave to rest for 5 minutes. Air-fry the chips at the same temperature for 16 minutes.

KCAL	CARBS	PROTEIN	FAT		
497	44g	34g	20g		

STEAK WITH CHIMICHURRI AND CUBED PAPRIKA POTATOES

SERVES: 2 | **PREP**: 5 MINS | **COOK**: 15–20 MINS | GF + DF + NF

Chimichurri tastes so delicious I think I could drink it, and with steak it's the ultimate combo. Teamed with cubed potatoes spiced with paprika, it's heaven in your mouth.

2 medium potatoes,
cut into 2.5cm cubes

Low-calorie
cooking spray

2 tsp paprika

2 lean rib-eye
steaks (360g)

2 tsp olive oil

Salt and pepper

Chimichurri

1 tbsp extra virgin
olive oil

2 tbsp finely chopped
fresh parsley

2 slices of red onion,
finely diced

1 tsp red wine vinegar

1 small red chilli,
finely diced

2 garlic cloves, minced

Squeeze of lemon juice

Side suggestion
Side salad

Swap: Choose your favourite steak cut for this recipe.

TIP: *If you can spare the calories, add another tablespoon or two of olive oil to the chimichurri to make it go further.*

Preheat the oven to 180°C.

Spray the cubed potatoes with low-calorie cooking spray and season with salt, pepper and the paprika. Place on a lined baking tray and cook in the oven for 15–20 minutes, flipping halfway, and spraying with more low-calorie cooking spray.

Meanwhile, in a small bowl, mix the chimichurri ingredients together and set aside. Season the steaks with salt, pepper and the 2 teaspoons of olive oil. Heat a griddle or frying pan on a high heat, then fry the steaks for about 2 minutes a side (if you like it medium-rare like me!). Leave to rest for a couple of minutes.

Slice the steaks, place on top of the paprika cubed potatoes and drizzle over the chimichurri to serve.

Air fryer method: Air-fry the seasoned cubed potatoes that you've sprayed with low-calorie cooking spray at 200°C for 14–18 mins. Turn halfway through cooking and spray with more low-calorie cooking spray.

KCAL	CARBS	PROTEIN	FAT		
487	41g	48g	15g		

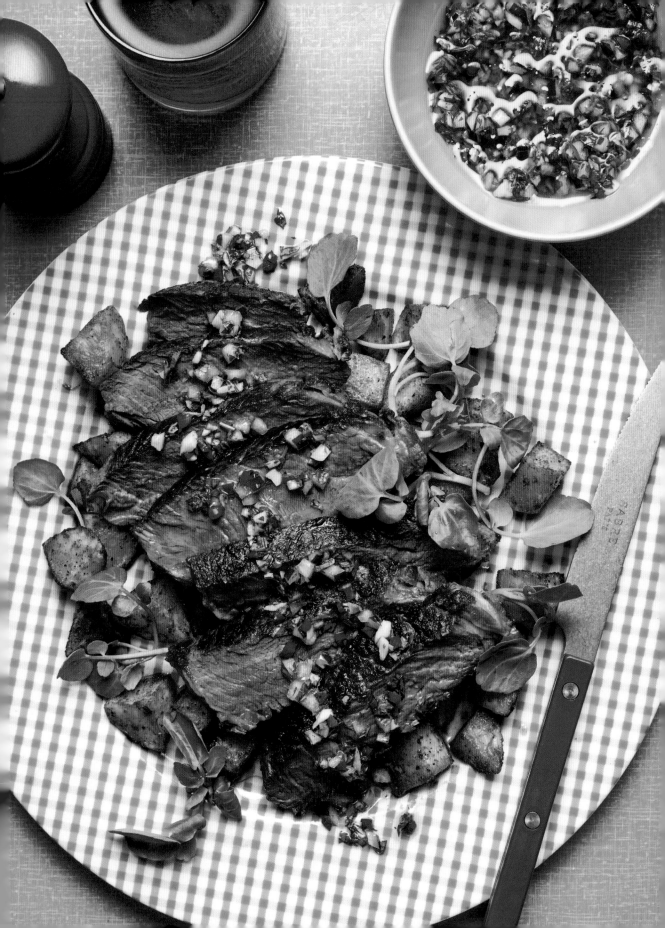

CUBANOS

SERVES: 2 | **PREP**: 2 MINS | **COOK**: 8–10 MINS | GF + NF

If you like gherkins and mustard, this sandwich is for you. A Cubano is a Cuban sandwich traditionally filled with roasted pork, Swiss cheese, pickles and mustard, but I have made a few changes to keep the calories low and to amplify the flavour.

4 slices of oak-smoked ham

4 slices of pork loin

2 gluten-free ciabatta rolls

1 tbsp low-fat butter, melted

1 tsp Dijon or English mustard

2 gherkins, thinly sliced

40g reduced-fat Cheddar, sliced

40g reduced-fat mozzarella, sliced

Side suggestions

Side salad

Low-calorie salted crisps

Swaps: If you can't find sliced pork loin, any pork slices will do, or you can swap the pork for sliced chicken.

Fry the smoked ham and pork loin in a hot pan for a few minutes to char.

Slice the ciabatta rolls in half and spread over the melted butter on the outside. On the inside halves, spread over the mustard (add more if you want it spicier), then add the sliced gherkins, meat slices and cheeses.

Cook for 3–4 minutes in a panini grill, under a standard grill, or in the same pan that you used for cooking the meat with parchment paper on top of the sandwich and something heavy to weight the Cubanos down. Make sure to flip them and cook on both sides. Serve.

KCAL	CARBS	PROTEIN	FAT
342	24g	28g	14g

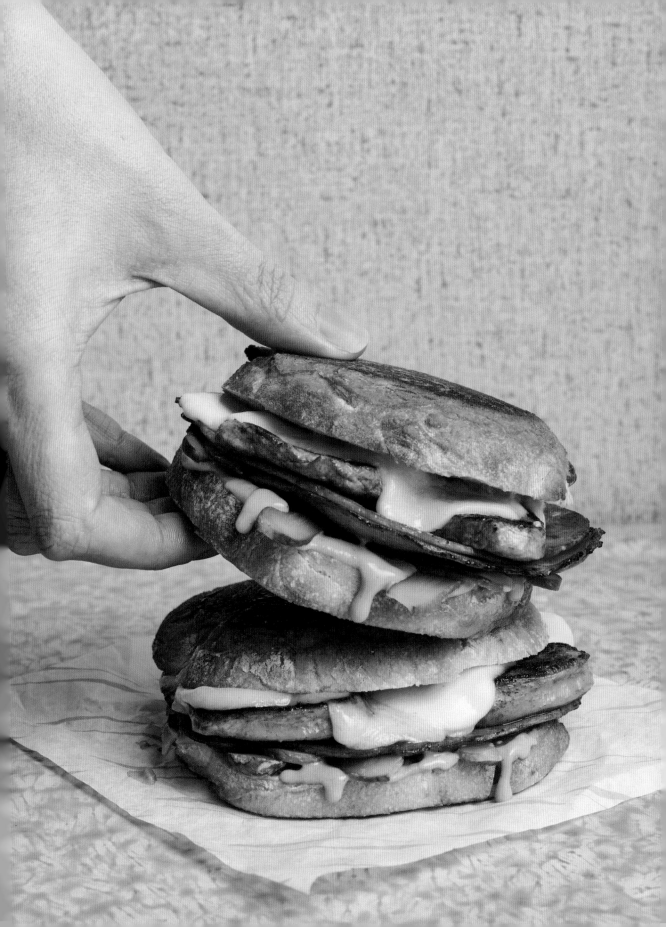

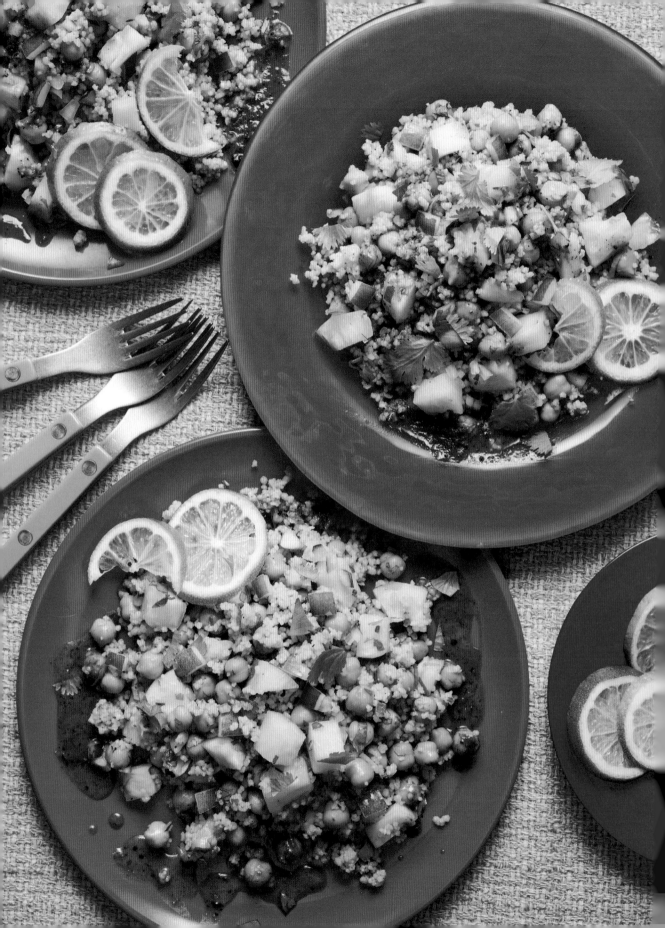

JERK AND COCONUT CHICKPEAS WITH PINEAPPLE COUSCOUS

SERVES: 2 | **PREP:** 5 MINS | **COOK:** 6–7 MINS | VE + DF + NF

Spicy jerk marinade with creamy coconut milk, served with
a zesty pineapple salsa to cool your taste buds.

400g tin chickpeas,
    drained
1 tbsp jerk marinade
50g reduced-fat
    coconut milk

Pineapple couscous
100g dried couscous
200ml hot vegetable
    stock
300g fresh
    pineapple, diced
¼ red onion,
    finely diced
3–4 tbsp finely
    chopped fresh
    coriander
Juice of ½ lime

Add the chickpeas to a pan along with the jerk marinade
and coconut milk. Mix well and cook on a medium heat for
6–7 minutes.

Meanwhile, place the couscous in a bowl and pour over the
vegetable stock, mixing well. Place a plate over the top and
let it steam for 6–7 minutes.

In a large bowl, mix the pineapple, red onion, coriander and
lime juice together, then add the couscous and serve with the
jerk chickpeas.

TIP: *Add less
jerk marinade
if you don't like
it too spicy.*

KCAL	CARBS	PROTEIN	FAT
435	80g	17g	8g

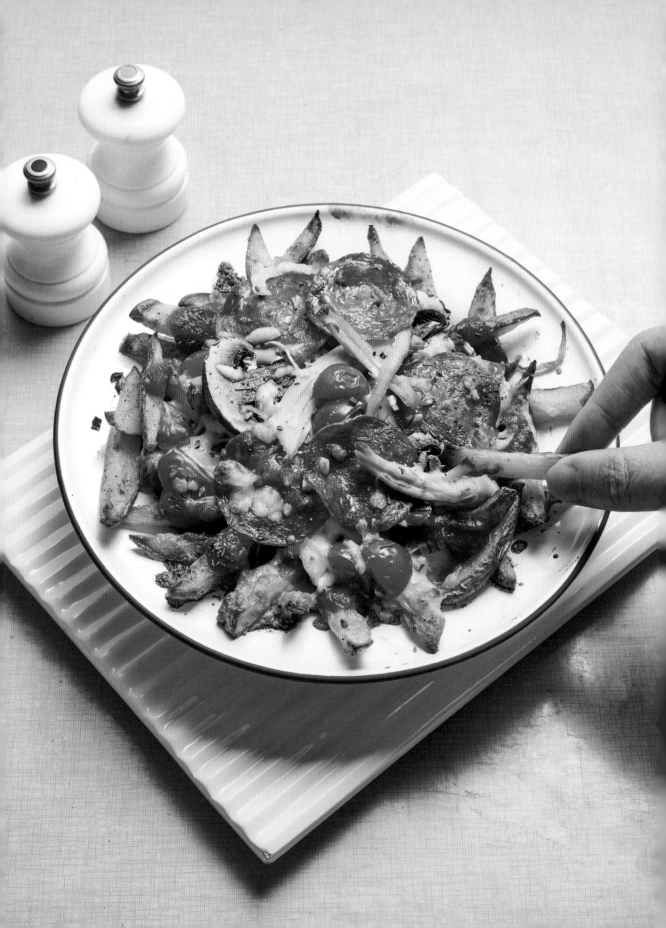

PIZZA-LOADED FRIES

SERVES: 2 | **PREP:** 5 MINS | **COOK:** 21–23 MINS | GF + NF

I'm here for anything with pizza flavours, so just imagine all the flavours of a pizza on a bed of homemade fries, which you can customise with your best pizza toppings. Get in my belly.

2 medium potatoes,
   cut into fries
Low-calorie
   cooking spray
1 tsp paprika
150g cooked chicken,
   shredded
2–3 mushrooms,
   finely sliced
3–4 cherry tomatoes,
   quartered
1–2 slices of red
   onion, finely diced
50g reduced-fat
   mozzarella, shredded
30g pepperoni slices
Salt and pepper

Marinara sauce
100g passata
20g tomato purée
1 tsp dried oregano

**Swaps: Choose
whatever toppings
you'd like – go wild!**

Mix the marinara sauce ingredients together and set aside.

Preheat the oven to 200°C.

Place the fries on a lined baking tray, then spray with plenty of low-calorie cooking spray and season with salt, pepper and the paprika, making sure they're evenly coated. Cook for 16–18 minutes, flipping halfway. Top with the homemade marinara sauce and the toppings in any order you fancy and cook for a further 5 minutes.

Air fryer method: Air-fry the fries at 200°C for 15 minutes, flipping halfway. Transfer the fries to a large sheet of foil, top with the marinara sauce, chicken, veg, cheese and pepperoni slices, then air-fry for a further 3–4 minutes. Alternatively, transfer the fries to 2 ovenproof dishes, add the toppings and air-fry separately for 3–4 minutes each.

KCAL	CARBS	PROTEIN	FAT		
401	44g	30g	12g	❄	

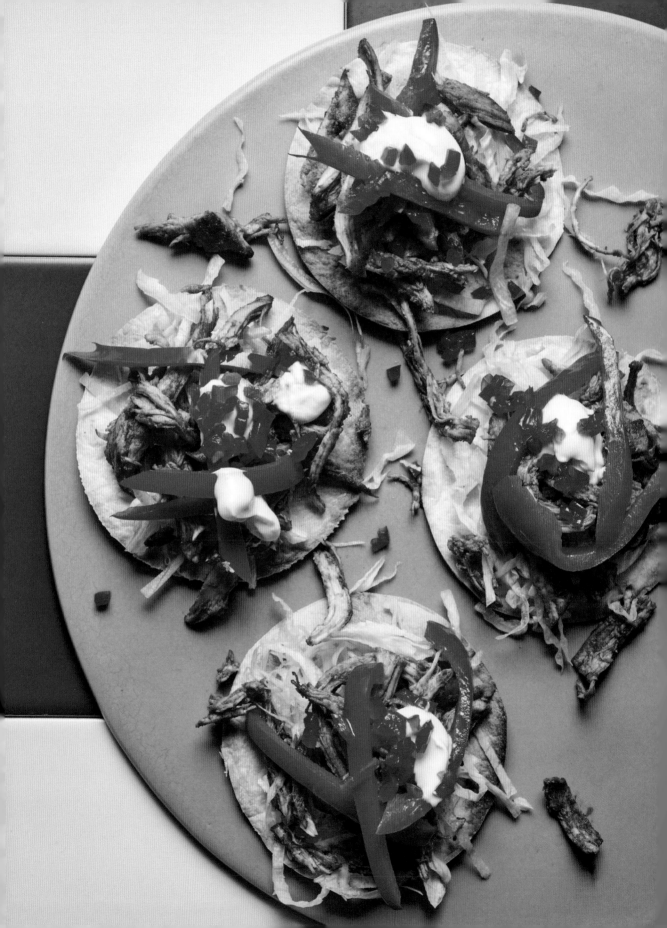

SMOKY PULLED CHICKEN TOSTADAS

SERVES: 2 | PREP: 2 MINS | COOK: 10–12 MINS | NF

A super quick recipe if you're shattered after work or for a speedy lunch. Tostadas are usually deep-fried in oil to get the tortilla super crispy, but we don't want to be drenched in oil now, do we?

4 mini tortilla wraps

2 chicken breasts, diced

2 tsp smoked paprika

Pinch of salt

Low-calorie cooking spray

1 red pepper, sliced

2 tbsp water

2 tbsp tomato purée

4 handfuls of iceberg lettuce, sliced

10 cherry tomatoes, finely diced

4 tbsp reduced-fat soured cream

Preheat the oven to 180°C.

Oven-cook the mini tortilla wraps for 3–5 minutes until crispy, then set aside.

Season the diced chicken with the paprika and salt. Spray a frying pan with low-calorie cooking spray and fry the chicken for 5–6 minutes or until cooked. Remove from the pan and set aside. Spray the same pan with more low-calorie cooking spray and fry the red pepper for a few minutes to soften. While the pepper is softening, shred the cooked chicken using two forks.

Add the chicken back to the pan, then pour in the water and tomato purée and mix well for 30–60 seconds or until everything goes lovely and sticky.

Place a handful of lettuce on top of each mini tortilla and top with the pulled chicken and peppers, and a tablespoon of soured cream.

Air fryer method: Place the mini tortilla wraps in the air fryer at 200°C for a couple of minutes to crisp up. (You may need to place a small bowl on top of the tortillas, so they don't fly away in the air fryer.)

KCAL	CARBS	PROTEIN	FAT		
456	44g	50g	9g		

PEANUT PORK WRAPS WITH EYE-POPPIN' SLAW

SERVES: 2 | **PREP**:5 MINS (+30 MINS MARINATING) | **COOK**: 6 MINS | DF

This is probably the best wrap I've ever made. Satay-style pork with a zingy slaw and a lovely crunch of peanuts. When I tell you that the flavours dance in your mouth and have a party, they really do.

2 lean pork steaks (400g)

1 heaped tbsp peanut butter

1 tsp soy sauce

1 tsp granulated or powdered sweetener

4–5 tbsp water

Low-calorie cooking spray

2 tortilla wraps

Crushed peanuts (optional)

Eye-poppin' slaw

2.5cm piece of cucumber, sliced

2 slices of red onion

1 carrot, grated

40g red cabbage, grated

1 spring onion, finely sliced

Juice of ½ lime

Marinade

1 tsp soy sauce

1 tsp chilli powder

½ tsp garlic granules

½ tsp onion granules

Juice of ½ lime

1 tsp honey

Salt and pepper

Mix all the marinade ingredients together in a bowl and add the pork steaks. Leave to marinate for at least 30 minutes or overnight for a more intense flavour.

In a bowl, mix all the slaw ingredients together and set aside.

In a small bowl, mix the peanut butter with the soy sauce, sweetener and water – add the water a tablespoon at a time to get your desired consistency; I like mine slightly runny. Set aside.

Fry the pork steaks in low-calorie cooking spray on a high heat for 3 minutes on each side, then remove from the pan and leave to rest for 4 minutes. After this time, check to make sure they are cooked through, then dice.

Discard any juices from the slaw, then grab a wrap, add a handful of the slaw, half the diced pork, drizzle over the peanut sauce and add some crushed peanuts (if using). Wrap, then repeat to make the second wrap. Slice in half and enjoy!

Optional: Add some crushed peanuts for a crunchy peanut hit!

Air fryer method: Air-fry the pork steaks at 200°C for 6–7 minutes on each side.

Swap: Don't eat pork? Swap it for chicken or tofu instead.

KCAL	CARBS	PROTEIN	FAT		
486	34g	36g	14g	❄	

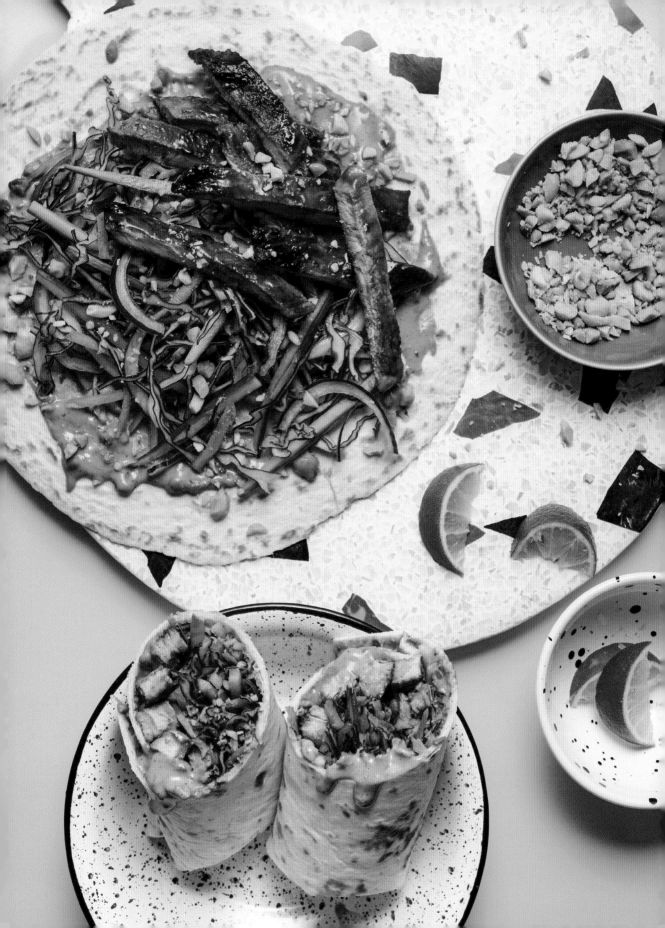

PASTA HEAVEN

SPINACH AND MUSHROOM CANNELLONI

SERVES: 4 | **PREP:** 10 MINS | **COOK:** 28–30 MINS | NF

I can't believe how tasty this meat-free recipe is and I don't even miss the meat. I must also admit, it tastes even better the next day.

240g baby spinach

Low-calorie
  cooking spray

1 medium onion,
  finely diced

250g mushrooms,
  finely diced

50ml vegetable stock

4 tbsp reduced-fat
  crème fraîche

½ tsp black pepper

170g cannelloni

500g passata

1 tsp dried oregano

80g reduced-fat
  Cheddar, grated

20g Parmesan, grated

Swaps: Don't fancy crème fraîche? Swap it for ricotta or light cream cheese and swap the Parmesan for a veggie version to make this vegetarian.

TIP: *If it's too hot, I leave the mixture for a few minutes before filling the cannelloni*

Preheat the oven to 200°C.

Add the spinach to a large bowl, then cover with boiling water and set aside.

Meanwhile, spray a large frying pan with low-calorie cooking spray and fry the onion and mushrooms for 3–4 minutes to soften. Drain the spinach, making sure you remove the excess water, and finely dice. Remove the pan from the heat and mix in the vegetable stock, crème fraîche, spinach and black pepper.

Now fill each cannelloni with the vegetable mixture – the easiest way to do this is to use a teaspoon to scoop the filling to the top of the cannelloni, then using the long handle of the spoon to push the mixture in. Transfer the filled cannelloni to a large ovenproof dish.

Next, pour over the passata and season with the oregano, carefully mixing it together (or do this in a bowl before pouring it over the cannelloni). Place a large sheet of foil over the top and enclose. Bake in the oven for 22–24 minutes or until the pasta is cooked.

Remove the foil, then sprinkle over all the grated cheese. Either stick it back in the oven until the cheese has melted or I like to speed things up by placing it under a hot grill for a few minutes.

KCAL	CARBS	PROTEIN	FAT	❄
317	40g	19g	8g	

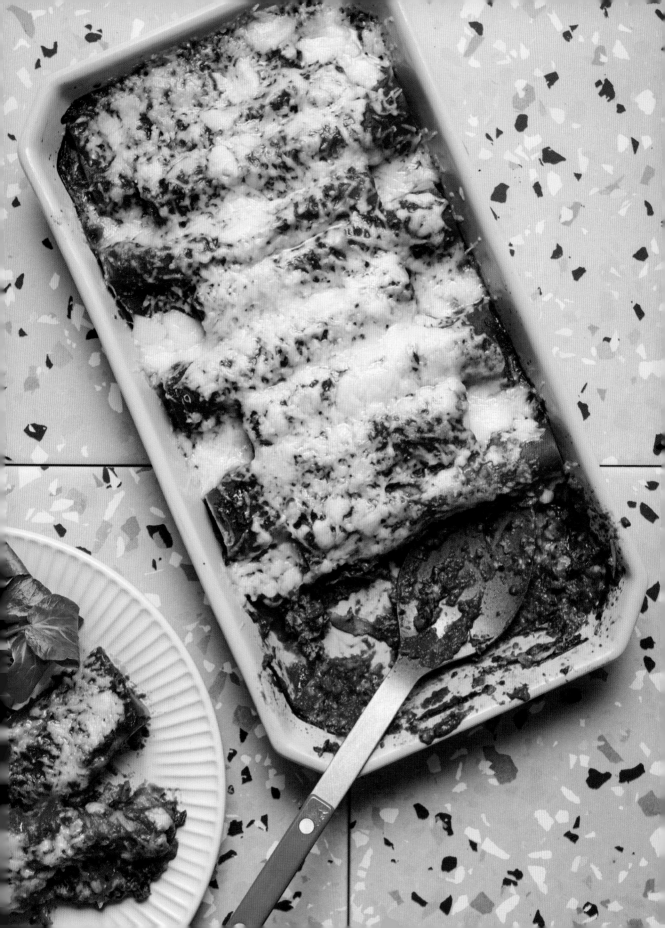

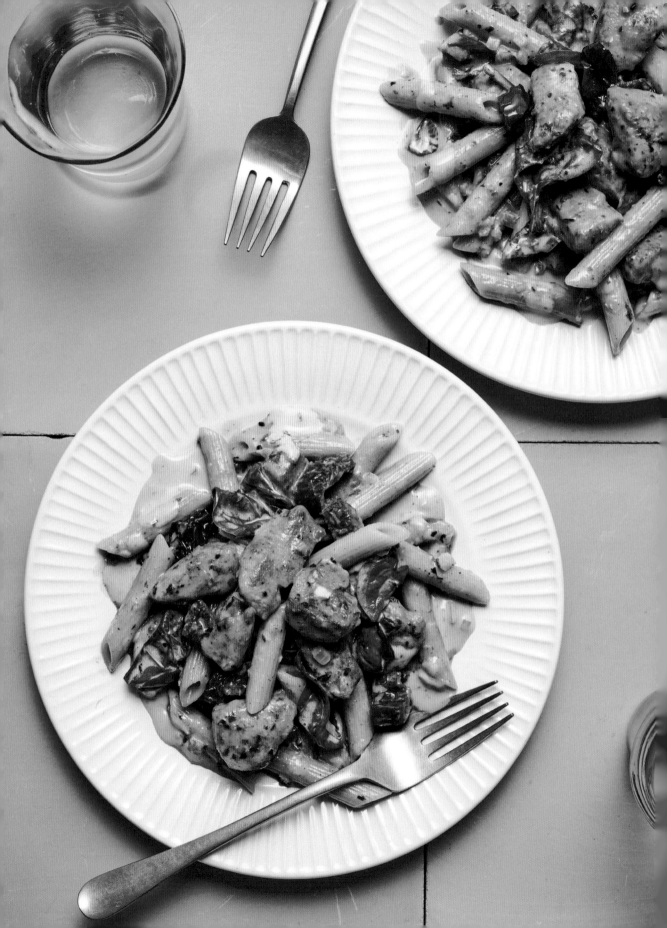

TUSCAN PASTA

SERVES: 2 | PREP: 2 MINS | COOK: 17–23 MINS | NF

Originating from the region of Tuscany in Italy, I cannot get enough of the flavours in this dish. A creamy, seasoned-to-perfection Parmesan sauce with sun-dried tomatoes, spinach and the tastiest chicken you could eat on its own. I guarantee this will become a staple in your house.

Low-calorie cooking spray

2 chicken breasts, diced

2 tsp Italian herbs

2 tsp smoked paprika

2 pinches of chilli flakes

20g Parmesan, grated

½ medium onion, finely diced

1 garlic clove, minced

100g dried penne pasta

400ml chicken stock

25g sun-dried tomatoes, sliced

1 tsp wholegrain mustard (or any will work!)

2 handfuls of spinach

50ml reduced-fat crème fraîche

Salt and pepper

Spray a large frying pan with low-calorie cooking spray, then add the diced chicken, season with 1 teaspoon of the Italian herbs, 1 teaspoon of the smoked paprika, a pinch of chilli flakes and some salt and pepper. Mix well and fry on a medium heat for 6–7 minutes. Sprinkle over the Parmesan cheese and stir well so that all the chicken is well coated, then fry for a further minute. Remove from the pan and set aside.

In the same pan, fry the onion with the garlic and remaining Italian herbs, paprika and chilli flakes. Use more low-calorie cooking spray if needed.

Add the pasta and then the chicken stock (starting with 300ml) and cook for 10–15 minutes until the stock has been absorbed and the pasta is cooked. Add the remaining 100ml stock if needed.

Stir in the sun-dried tomatoes, mustard, spinach, crème fraîche and the cooked chicken and enjoy!

Optional: Swap the low-calorie cooking spray for 1-2 teaspoons of the sun-dried tomato oil for added flavour.

KCAL	CARBS	PROTEIN	FAT	
499	45g	52g	12g	❄

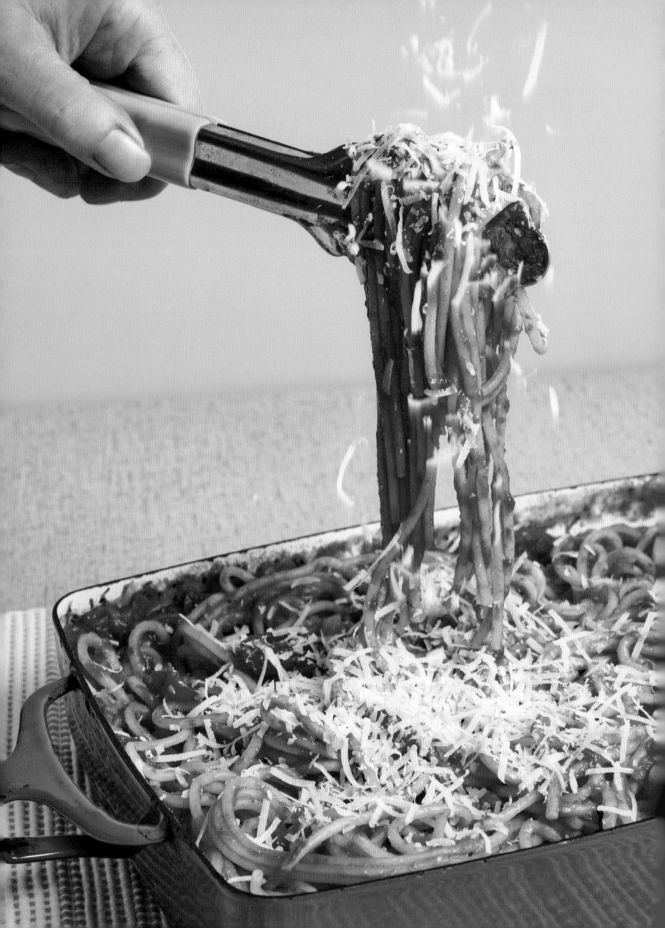

OVEN-BAKED SPAGHETTI

SERVES: 4 | **PREP:** 5 MINS | **COOK:** 25–30 MINS | NF

This recipe is inspired by a video I saw on TikTok that went viral and I knew I had to recreate it. Spaghetti cooked in the oven may sound odd, but this one-pot wonder gives you so much flavour for minimum effort.

230g spaghetti

1 onion, finely diced

2 garlic cloves, minced

150g cherry tomatoes, sliced

2 x 400g tins chopped tomatoes

2 tsp Italian herbs

370ml boiling water

4 tbsp Parmesan cheese, grated

10 basil leaves, torn

Salt and pepper

Side suggestion
Garlic bread

Swap: To make this veggie, swap the Parmesan for a veggie version!

Preheat the oven to 200°C.

Chuck all the ingredients, apart from the Parmesan cheese and a few basil leaves, into a large ovenproof dish and carefully give them a good mix.

Cover the dish with foil and bake in the oven for 15 minutes. Remove from the oven and mix well, then re-cover with the foil and cook for a further 10–15 minutes or until the pasta is cooked through.

Serve with the remaining torn basil leaves and a tablespoon of Parmesan per serving.

KCAL	CARBS	PROTEIN	FAT	
302	55g	12g	5g	

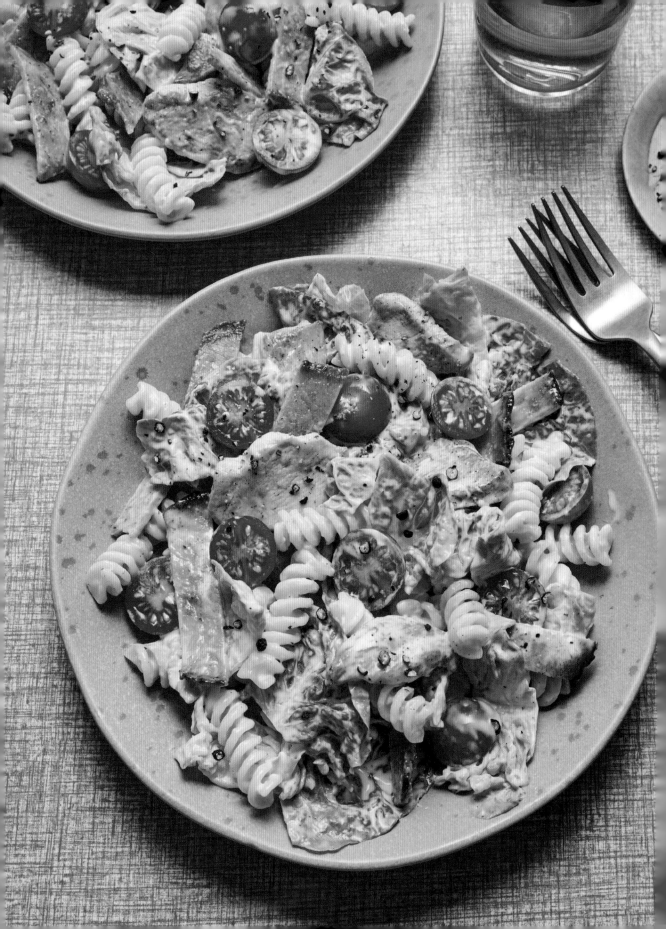

BLT CHICKEN PASTA SALAD

SERVES: 2 | **PREP:** 2 MINS | **COOK:** 8–10 MINS | DF + NF

You won't have had a pasta salad like this. If you're a big fan of a BLT sandwich like me, it tastes just like it but without the bread and plenty of protein to fill you up.

Low-calorie cooking spray

4 smoked bacon medallions, sliced

200g chicken breast, sliced

6 tbsp light mayonnaise

½ tsp garlic granules

100g dried pasta, cooked

10 cherry tomatoes, sliced

2 handfuls of romaine lettuce, sliced

Salt and pepper

Swap: If you don't mind extra calories, swap the bacon medallions for bacon rashers.

Spray a pan with low-calorie cooking spray and fry the bacon for 3–4 minutes. Remove from the pan and set aside. In the same pan, fry the sliced chicken with a pinch of salt and pepper for 5–6 minutes or until cooked.

In a small bowl, mix together the mayonnaise, another pinch of salt and pepper and the garlic granules.

Add the cooked pasta, cherry tomatoes and lettuce to a large bowl, then mix in the dressing. Top with the sliced chicken and bacon and serve.

KCAL	CARBS	PROTEIN	FAT	
467	47g	55g	7g	

CHICKEN SAUSAGE AND 'NDUJA RAGÙ

SERVES: 4 | **PREP**: 5 MINS | **COOK**: 13–18 MINS | DF + NF

Now I know ragù is meant to be slow-cooked but I'm all about quick recipes that don't compromise on flavour. I've added 'nduja to the ragù for a slightly spicy pork twist and chicken sausages to boost the protein content.

200g dried tagliatelle

Low-calorie cooking spray

½ onion, finely diced

1 celery stick, finely diced

1 medium carrot, finely diced

16 chicken sausages

2–3 garlic cloves, minced

2 tbsp 'nduja

500g passata

1 tsp dried thyme

Salt

Side suggestion

Garlic bread

Swaps: Swap the chicken sausages for pork or veggie sausages, and any pasta would work here.

Cook the tagliatelle in boiling salted water according to the packet instructions. Drain, then set aside, reserving a ladle of pasta water.

Meanwhile, spray a large frying pan with plenty of low-calorie cooking spray and fry the onion, celery and carrot for 3–4 minutes to soften. (I like to add a dash of water to help soften them, too.)

Skin the chicken sausages and fry alongside the veg, adding the garlic for a few minutes, and using a spatula to break apart the meat.

Mix in the 'nduja with a dash of water to loosen it, then add the passata and thyme. Reduce the sauce on a medium–high heat for 5–10 minutes, then mix in the cooked tagliatelle with a dash of the pasta water.

KCAL	CARBS	PROTEIN	FAT	
377	45g	28g	8g	

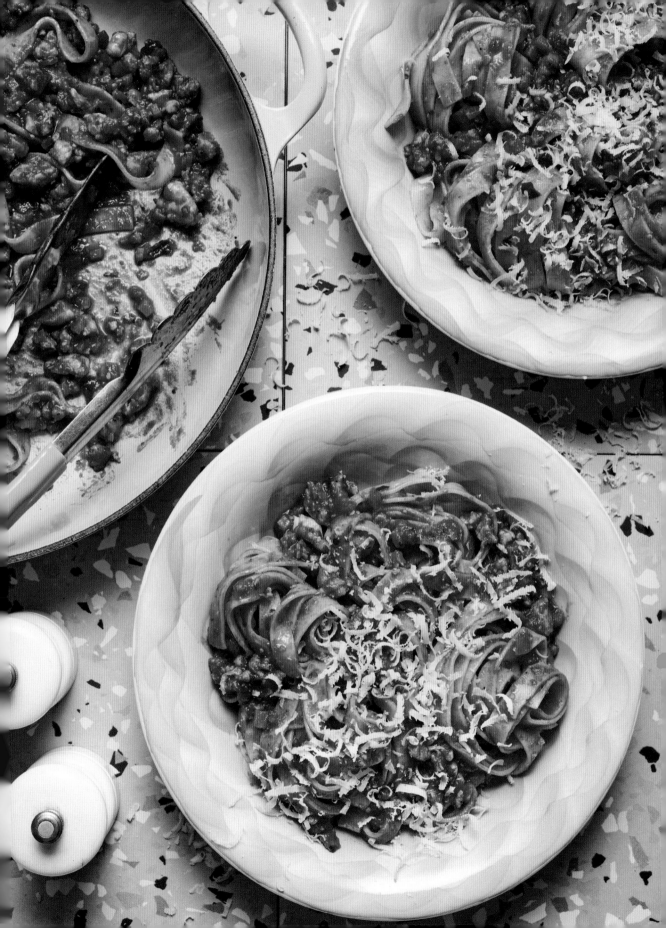

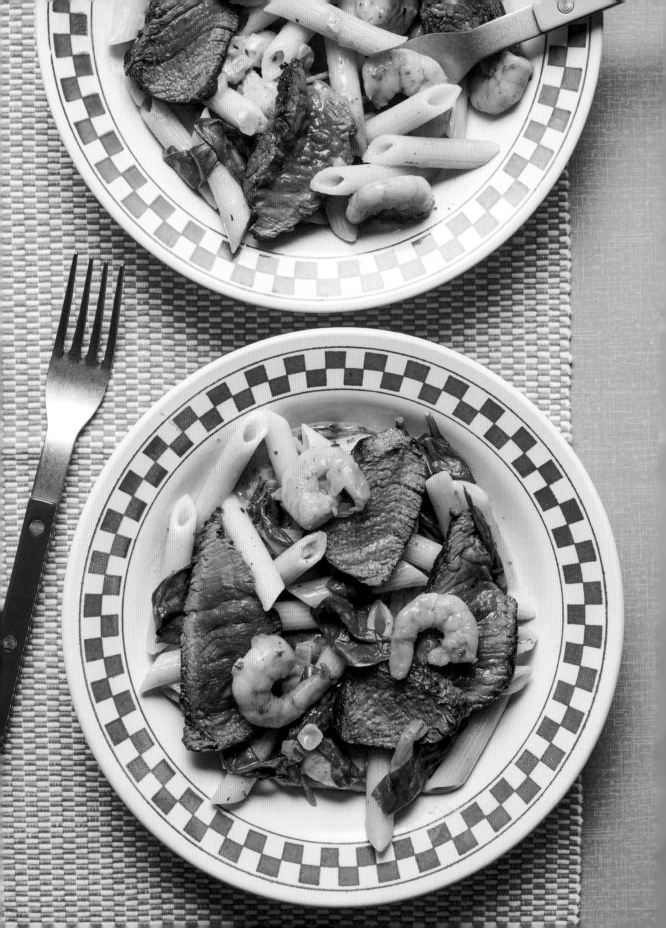

SURF AND TURF PASTA

SERVES: 2 | **PREP:** 2 MINS | **COOK:** 12–14 MINS | NF

I don't think you will have ever tried a pasta dish quite like this. Tender pieces of steak with wonderfully seasoned king prawns in a silky pasta sauce.

100g dried pasta
(any shape)

1 rump steak, fat
removed (230g)

Low-calorie
cooking spray

12 raw king prawns,
shelled and deveined

1½ tsp Cajun
seasoning

½ onion, finely diced

150ml vegetable stock

60g reduced-fat
crème fraîche

2 tbsp grated
Parmesan

A handful of spinach

1–2 tsp granulated
or powdered
sweetener (optional)

Salt and pepper

> **TIP:** *Use a good-quality steak as you'll really notice the difference in flavour.*

Cook the pasta in boiling salted water according to the packet instructions. Drain, then set aside, reserving 1–2 tablespoons of pasta water.

Meanwhile, season the steak with salt, pepper and a good spritz of low-calorie cooking spray (or use olive oil), rubbing in well. Fry in a hot, dry pan on a high heat for 2 minutes on each side. Remove from the pan and set aside to rest for 4 minutes.

Spray the same pan with low-calorie cooking spray. Season the prawns with 1 teaspoon of the Cajun seasoning and fry for 3–4 minutes on a medium heat or until cooked. Remove from the pan and set aside.

Spray the pan with more low-calorie cooking spray and fry the onion for 2–3 minutes to soften, then add the vegetable stock, crème fraîche, remaining ½ teaspoon of Cajun seasoning and the Parmesan, mixing well.

Simmer on a low heat for 2–3 minutes, then add the prawns, pasta, reserved pasta water and spinach. Keep stirring until the spinach has wilted, then plate up. Finished with the sliced steak.

Optional: If it tastes too salty, add 1-2 teaspoons of sweetener.

KCAL	CARBS	PROTEIN	FAT	
487	45g	45g	14g	❄

BUFFALO CHICKEN MAC AND CHEESE

SERVES: 2 | **PREP:** 2 MINS | **COOK:** 12 MINS | NF

Whoever created mac and cheese is a hero. I decided to change it up by adding my favourite sauce in the world, hot sauce, to the mix. But don't worry, the creamy mac and cheese cools down the heat from the hot sauce perfectly and if you still want a big flavour kick, just add more hot sauce.

100g dried macaroni

2 chicken breasts, diced

½ tsp garlic granules

1 tsp paprika

Low-calorie cooking spray

2 tbsp buffalo sauce

40g reduced-fat mozzarella, grated (optional)

Salt and pepper

Cheese sauce

40g light soft cheese

60g reduced-fat Cheddar, grated

50ml semi-skimmed milk

Side suggestions

Side salad

Coleslaw

Cook the pasta in boiling salted water according to the packet instructions. Drain, then set aside, reserving 1 tablespoon of pasta water.

Meanwhile, season the diced chicken with the garlic granules, paprika and some salt and pepper. Spray a frying pan with low-calorie spray and cook the chicken on a medium heat for 5–6 minutes. Remove the chicken from the pan and leave to rest for a few minutes. Dice into smaller chunks, then mix it with 1½ tablespoons of the buffalo sauce.

Mix the cheese sauce ingredients into the cooked macaroni, along with the pasta water, until it turns lovely and creamy. Add a bit of heat if needed.

Mix in half the chicken until well combined, then top with the remaining chicken and ½ tablespoon of buffalo sauce.

Optional: Add some reduced-fat mozzarella at the end and melt under a hot grill for the best cheese pull.

Air fryer method: Spray the seasoned chicken with low-calorie cooking spray and air-fry at 200°C for 5–6 minutes or until cooked.

KCAL	CARBS	PROTEIN	FAT
443	41g	60g	5g

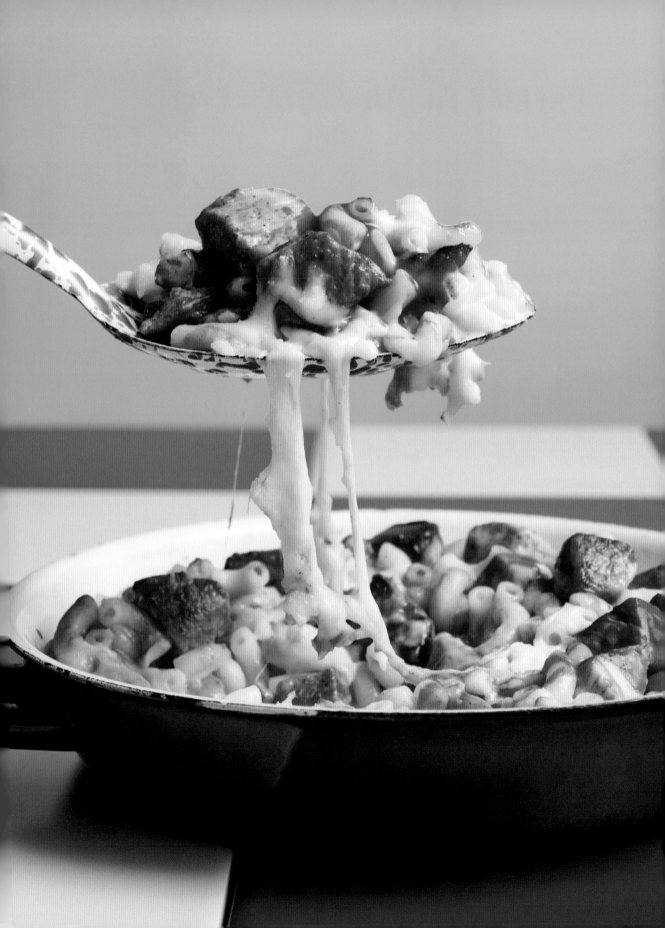

CREAMY FAJITA PASTA

SERVES: 2 | **PREP:** 2 MINS | **COOK:** 10–12 MINS | NF

This was one of my first recipes to go viral on TikTok and has had over 2 million views! It blew my mind and it's so simple to make you won't believe it.

100g dried pasta

2 chicken breasts, sliced

3 tsp fajita seasoning

Low-calorie cooking spray

1 red pepper, sliced

1 yellow pepper, sliced

¼ red onion, sliced

80g light soft cheese

Low-fat Cheddar, grated (optional)

Cook the pasta in boiling salted water according to the packet instructions. Drain, then set aside, reserving 3 tablespoons of pasta water.

Meanwhile, season the chicken with 2 teaspoons of fajita seasoning. Spray a frying pan with low-calorie cooking spray and fry the seasoned chicken slices for 3–4 minutes, then add the sliced veg and 1 tablespoon of pasta water and cook for a further 3–4 minutes.

Add the remaining 1 teaspoon of fajita seasoning, the soft cheese and remaining 2 tablespoons of pasta water. Mix well on a medium heat until it forms a creamy sauce, then mix in the cooked pasta. Coat the pasta well in the sauce and serve.

Optional: Low-fat grated Cheddar on top is a winner!

KCAL	CARBS	PROTEIN	FAT	
491	57g	53g	5g	

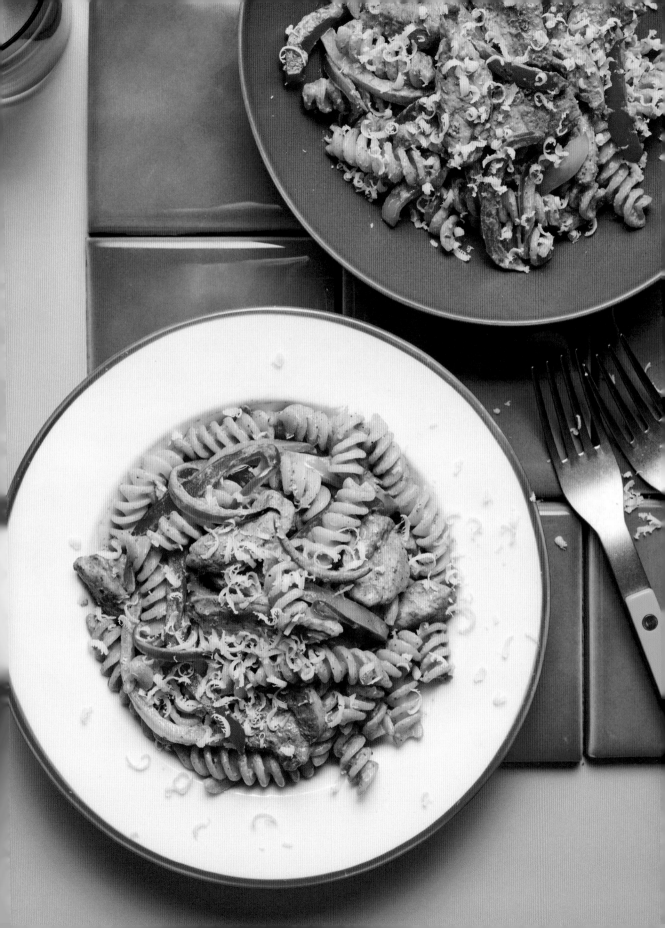

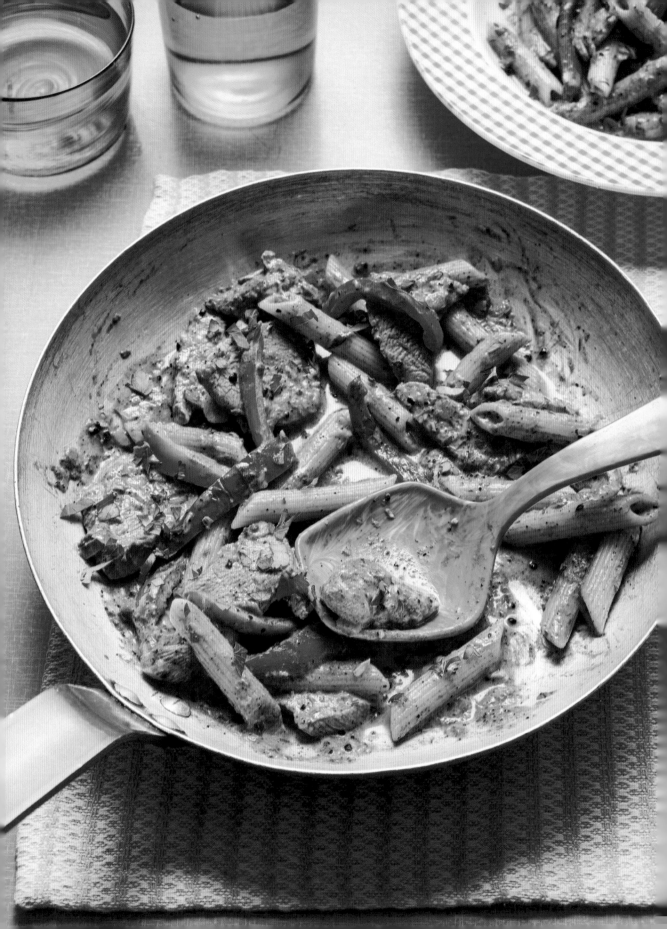

JAMAICAN-STYLE PASTA

SERVES: 2 | **PREP**: 5 MINS | **COOK**: 10–12 MINS | NF

If you love jerk flavours, then you've got to try this Jamaican pasta dish. It's a creamy pasta with colourful peppers and chicken, all infused with jerk seasoning. Comforting and spicy in all the right ways.

100g dried
  penne pasta
2 chicken breasts,
  sliced
3 tsp jerk seasoning
1 tbsp jerk marinade
Low-calorie
  cooking spray
½ onion, finely diced
½ red pepper, sliced
½ green pepper, sliced
60g reduced-fat
  crème fraîche
2–3 tbsp Parmesan
  cheese, grated
2–3 tbsp finely
  chopped fresh
  parsley
½ lime (optional)

Cook the pasta in boiling salted water according to the packet instructions. Drain, reserving 1–2 ladles of pasta water and set aside.

Marinate the chicken in 2 teaspoons of the jerk seasoning and the jerk marinade and set aside.

Spray a large frying pan with low-calorie cooking spray and fry the onion and peppers for a couple of minutes to soften. Move to one side of the pan, spray the empty side with more low-calorie cooking spray, then fry the chicken for 6–7 minutes until cooked.

Add the remaining 1 teaspoon of jerk seasoning to the veg, give it a mix, then combine everything together. Stir in the crème fraîche, with 1–2 ladles of the pasta water and the Parmesan cheese, then mix in the pasta.

Finish with a sprinkle of parsley.

Optional: Try squeezing over ½ lime when serving to make it less spicy and give it a zesty hit!

KCAL	CARBS	PROTEIN	FAT	❄
496	48g	50g	11g	

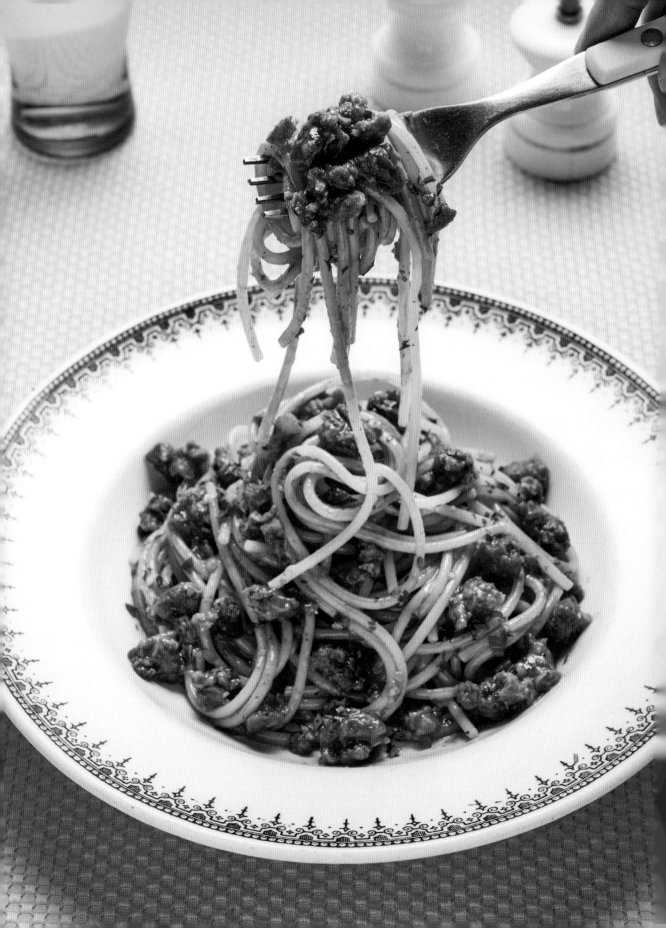

CHORIZONARA

SERVES: 2 | **PREP**: 2 MINS | **COOK**: 10 MINS | NF

To all the Italians out there – please look away now. I have used the traditional method of making a carbonara, but instead of using pancetta I swapped it for chorizo. Game changer!

100g dried spaghetti
90g chorizo, diced
2 egg yolks
4 tbsp grated
  Parmesan
½ tsp black pepper
1 tsp smoked paprika
Salt

To serve (optional)
Squeeze of lemon juice
Fresh parsley, chopped

Side suggestions
Tenderstem broccoli
Garlic bread

Cook the spaghetti in boiling salted water for 8–10 minutes or until cooked to your liking. Drain, then set aside, reserving a few tablespoons of pasta water.

Meanwhile, fry the diced chorizo for 3–4 minutes, using a little low-calorie cooking spray if needed, but the chorizo should release its own oils.

In a small bowl, mix together the egg yolks, Parmesan, black pepper and paprika until it forms a paste. Then mix in the pasta water.

Add the cooked pasta to the pan with the chorizo and mix well, then remove from the heat and mix in the egg mixture for about a minute. Serve and enjoy!

Optional: A squeeze of lemon juice and a sprinkle of fresh parsley cuts through the saltiness of this dish really well.

KCAL	CARBS	PROTEIN	FAT	
486	39g	23g	28g	❄

LASAGNE POCKETS

SERVES: 4 | **PREP**: 5 MINS | **COOK**: 25–30 MINS | NF

If you fancy a change from your usual lasagne recipe, then give these pockets a try. Yummy Bolognese sauce encased in lasagne sheets, with the easiest and tastiest béchamel sauce drenched over each pocket. Your whole family will love them!

Low-calorie
  cooking spray
½ onion, finely diced
½ red pepper,
  finely diced
8 mushrooms,
  finely diced
250g lean beef mince
400g tin chopped
  tomatoes
2 tbsp tomato purée
2 tsp mixed herbs
100ml beef stock
8 dried lasagne sheets

Béchamel
15g low-fat butter
15g plain flour
150ml semi-
  skimmed milk
50g reduced-fat
  Cheddar, grated

Side suggestions
Salad
Garlic bread

TIP: *I normally have beef mixture left over, which you can use for pasta sauce.*

Preheat the oven to 180°C.

Spray a large frying pan with low-calorie cooking spray and fry the onion, pepper and mushrooms for a few minutes to soften.

Add the beef mince and fry for a further few minutes, then mix in the chopped tomatoes, tomato purée, mixed herbs and beef stock. Simmer for 8 minutes or until the stock has reduced.

Meanwhile, pre-cook the lasagne sheets in boiling water for 5 minutes.

In a small pan, melt the butter, then mix in the flour until it forms a paste. On a low–medium heat, gradually whisk in the milk, a small amount at a time, until it starts to thicken.

Grab a pre-cooked lasagne sheet and place on a lined baking tray sprayed with low-calorie cooking spray. Place a second lasagne sheet over the top to form a cross, then add 1 tablespoon of béchamel in the middle, then a ladle of beef mixture.

Fold each end of the lasagne towards the centre of the cross until the filling is enclosed, then cover with béchamel and grated Cheddar. Repeat to make the other 3 pockets.

Bake for 15–18 minutes.

KCAL	CARBS	PROTEIN	FAT	❄️
356	43g	26g	9g	

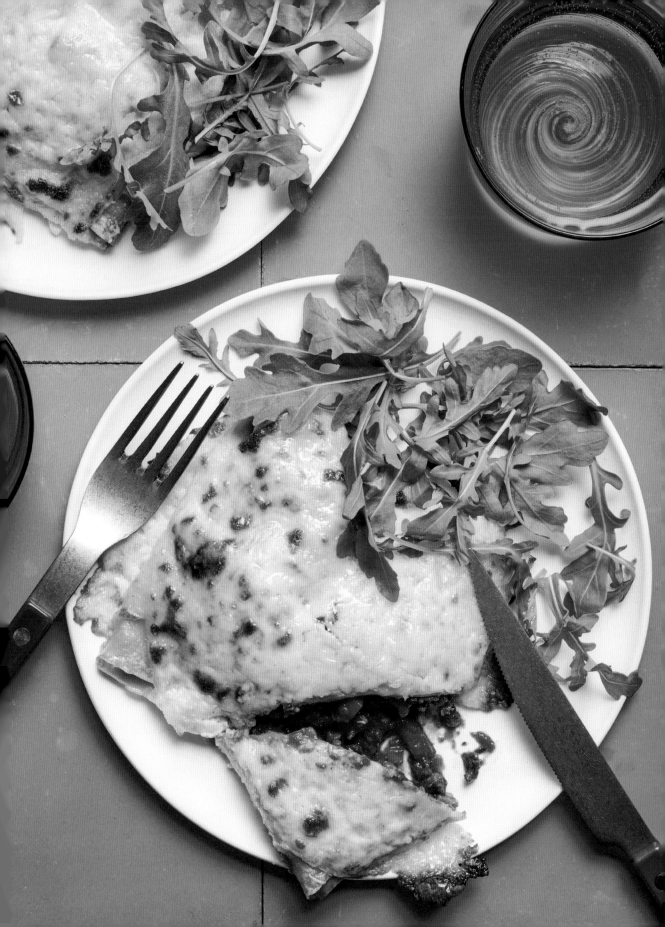

THE ULTIMATE HIDDEN VEG PASTA

SERVES: 4 | **PREP**: 5 MINS | **COOK**: 25–30 MINS | V + NF

Got any fussy eaters at home who don't like eating veg? All you need
to do is make this recipe. The sauce contains 5 out of your 5-a-day (yes,
REALLY) and you could even eat it as a soup, it's that tasty.

1 medium courgette,
  sliced

330g cherry or
  plum tomatoes

1 medium onion, diced

1 red pepper, diced

2 garlic cloves

1 tsp Italian
  mixed herbs

Low-calorie
  cooking spray

320g dried penne
  pasta

100g light soft cheese

100ml vegetable stock

Salt

Side suggestion
Garlic bread

Preheat the oven to 200°C.

Place all the veg and Italian mixed herbs in a large ovenproof
dish and spray with low-calorie cooking spray. Roast in the
oven for 25–30 minutes.

Meanwhile, cook the pasta in boiling salted water according
to the packet instructions. Drain, then set aside, reserving a
ladle of pasta water.

Add the roast veg to a blender along with the soft cheese
and vegetable stock and blend. If you prefer a thinner sauce,
add the ladle of reserved pasta water.

Mix the sauce with the cooked pasta and serve.

KCAL	CARBS	PROTEIN	FAT	
368	69g	15g	3g	❄

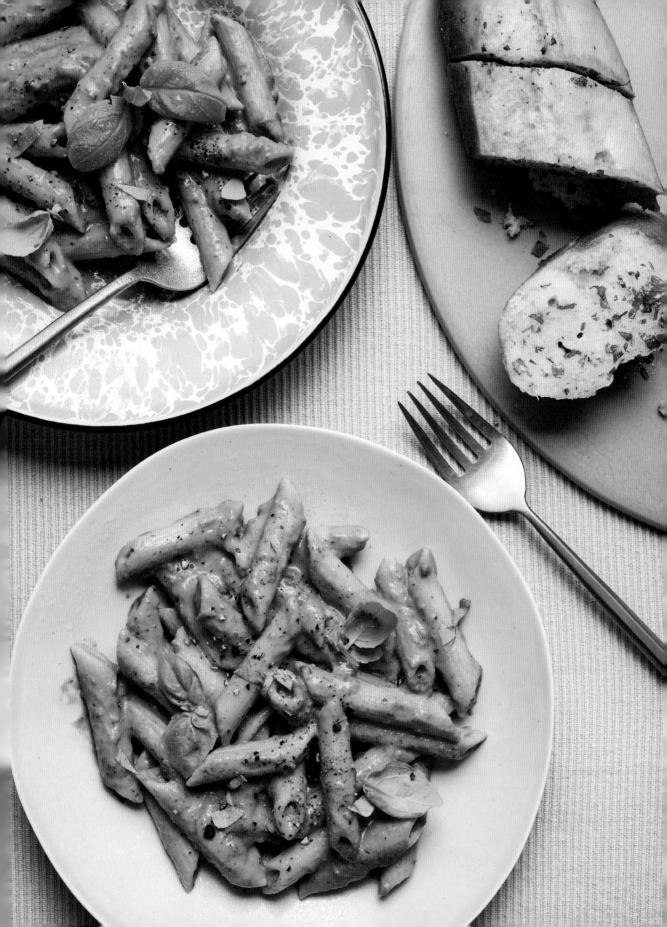

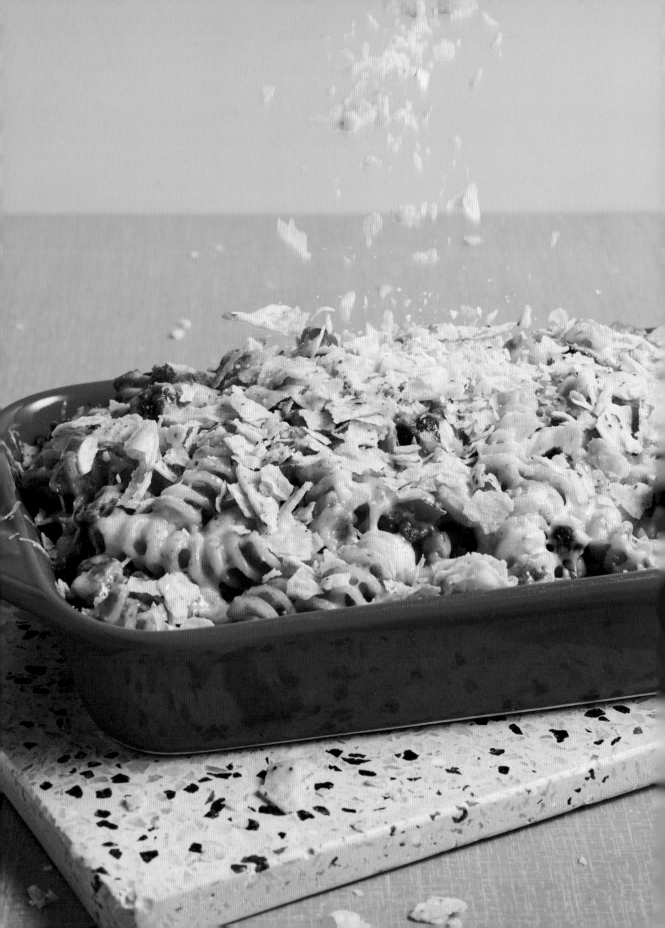

TEX MEX PASTA BAKE WITH TORTILLA CRUMB

SERVES: 4 | **PREP:** 5 MINS | **COOK:** 12–14 MINS | NF

A savoury, cheesy, Mexican-style pasta bake with a tortilla crumb for a texture sensation. It's the kind of satisfying, comforting pasta recipe that the whole family will love.

200g dried pasta
(any shape)

Low-calorie
cooking spray

½ onion, finely diced

1 red pepper,
finely diced

400g lean beef mince

2 tbsp taco seasoning

1 tbsp tomato purée

400g tin chopped
tomatoes

100g tinned sweetcorn

120g tinned red
kidney beans

100g reduced-fat
Cheddar, grated

25g lightly salted
tortilla chips

Salt and pepper

Cook the pasta in boiling salted water according to the packet instructions. Drain, then set aside, reserving a few tablespoons of pasta water.

Meanwhile, spray a large frying pan with low-calorie cooking spray and fry the onion for a few minutes to soften, then add the red pepper and beef mince. Fry for a further 4–5 minutes, making sure to break apart the mince with a spatula, then add the taco seasoning and tomato purée, mixing well.

Add the remaining ingredients, apart from the cheese and tortilla chips, and fry for a further few minutes. Mix in half of the cheese, then stir in the cooked pasta along with a dash of pasta water.

Transfer to a large ovenproof dish and add the remaining cheese. Place under a hot grill for a few minutes to melt the cheese.

Meanwhile, bash the tortilla chips into crumbs in a freezer bag or crumble with your hands. Remove the pasta bake from the oven and top with the crumbled tortilla chips.

KCAL	CARBS	PROTEIN	FAT	
491	58g	42g	9g	

ONE-POT WONDERS

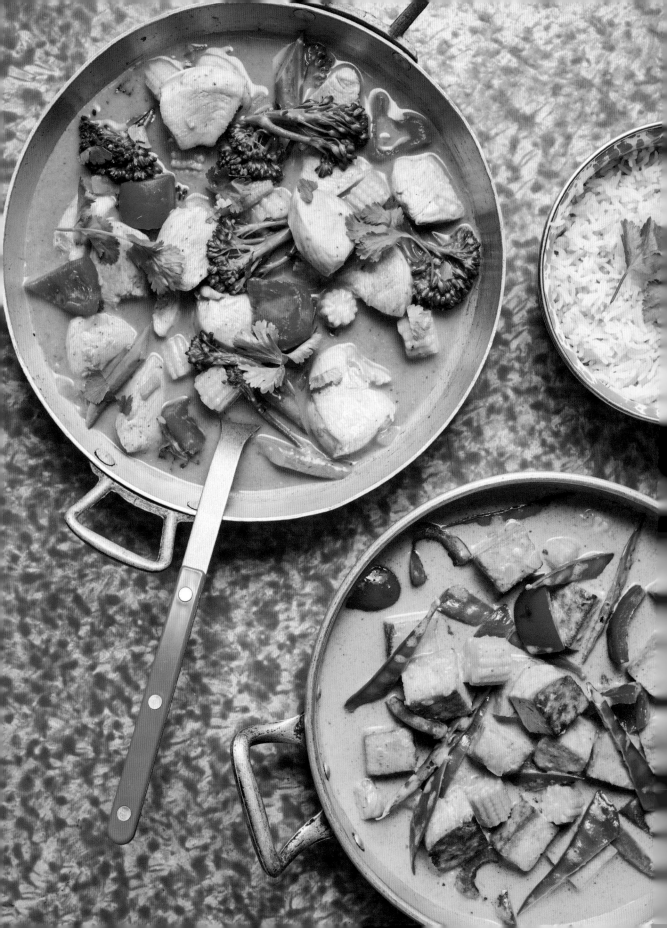

THAI CURRY TWO WAYS

SERVES: 2 | **PREP:** 2 MINS | **COOK:** 8–15 MINS | DF + NF

Here I've made a Thai Red Curry and a Thai Green Curry, although you'll see they are very similar to make. I always find that Thai food is bursting with such an amazing complexity of flavours, so it's one of my favourite cuisines when I eat out. But instead of paying an arm and a leg for a curry, make it at home faster than waiting for it at a restaurant. Bonus – it will taste exactly the same.

Low-calorie
   cooking spray
½ medium onion, diced
2 garlic cloves, minced
2.5cm piece of fresh
   ginger, peeled
   and minced
½ medium red
   pepper, diced
A handful of baby
   corn, sliced
200ml reduced-fat
   coconut milk
A few dashes of
   fish sauce
1 tsp granulated or
   powdered sweetener
1 tsp soy sauce
Coriander, to serve
   (optional)

Green curry
250g extra-firm
   tofu, cubed
50g Thai green
   curry paste
A handful of mangetout

Red curry
2 chicken breasts, diced
50g Thai red curry paste
A handful of Tenderstem
   broccoli, sliced

Side suggestion
Basmati rice

For both the green and red curry, in a large, lidded pan, fry the onion in low-calorie cooking spray for 2–3 minutes to soften, then add the garlic, ginger and tofu for the green curry, or chicken for the red curry.

For the green curry, fry for a further few minutes to fragrance the tofu, then mix in the Thai green curry paste, baby corn, red pepper and mangetout with 2–3 tablespoons of water to loosen. Fry for a minute, then pour in the coconut milk (mix it well before you pour it in), fish sauce, sweetener and soy sauce.

For the red curry, fry for 5–6 minutes, then mix in the red Thai curry paste, baby corn, red pepper and broccoli with 2–3 tablespoons of water to loosen. Fry for a minute, then pour in the coconut milk (mix it well before you pour it in), fish sauce, sweetener and soy sauce.

Simmer for 4–5 minutes with the lid on or until the veg is cooked to your liking and enjoy!

Optional: Top with coriander to serve.

Swaps: Swap in tofu, chicken, beef or prawns and swap the soy sauce for tamari to make this gluten-free.

Thai Green Curry	KCAL	CARBS	PROTEIN	FAT	❄️
	360	16g	21g	24g	

Thai Red Curry	KCAL	CARBS	PROTEIN	FAT	❄️
	401	16g	47g	17g	

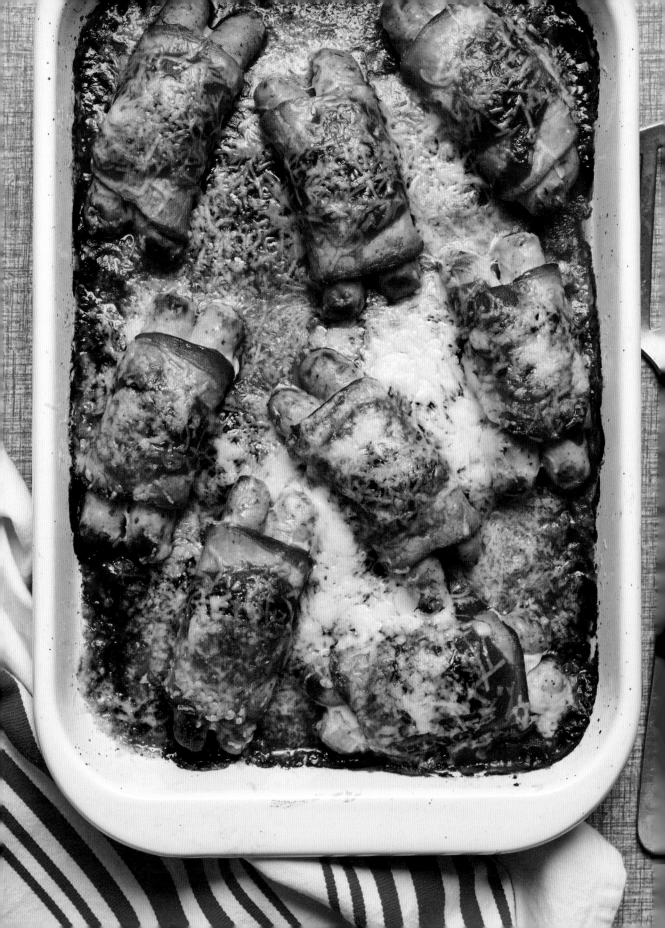

HUNTER'S CHICKEN SAUSAGES

SERVES: 4 | **PREP**: 5 MINS | **COOK**: 25–30 MINS | GF + NF

A nice change from your usual Hunter's chicken, my version uses bacon wrapped around chicken sausages with an irresistible sticky BBQ sauce. You can serve these with just about anything.

8 smoked bacon
    medallions

16 chicken sausages

100g passata

4 tbsp BBQ sauce

100g reduced-fat
    Cheddar, grated

Side suggestions

Mash and veg of
    your choice

Swaps: This recipe tastes great with pork or vegetarian sausages too. If you have a gluten intolerance check the sausages and BBQ sauce are both gluten-free.

Preheat the oven to 190°C.

Wrap each piece of bacon around 2 chicken sausages, then place in a large ovenproof dish and bake in the oven for 20 minutes.

Pour over the passata and spread over the BBQ sauce. Sprinkle over the grated Cheddar and return to the oven for a further 5–10 minutes and enjoy!

Air fryer method: Air-fry the bacon-wrapped sausages at 200°C for 8–10 minutes, then remove. (Cook in batches if necessary.) Place a sheet of foil in the air fryer, making sure it goes around the edges, then place the sausages in the foil, add the passata, BBQ sauce and grated Cheddar and air-fry for a further 5 minutes.

KCAL	CARBS	PROTEIN	FAT		
253	10g	41g	5g		

LEFTOVER PHO

SERVES: 4 | **PREP**: 2 MINS | **COOK**: 22–25 MINS | GF + DF + NF

This Vietnamese noodle soup is perfect when you have leftover meat from a roast lying about like roast chicken or beef. This soup is as fragrant as they come . . .

200g rice noodles

4 tsp chilli oil (optional)

Base

1 small onion, halved

2.5 litres chicken stock, made with 2 chicken stockpots or cubes

5cm piece of fresh ginger, sliced

2 star anise

1 tbsp granulated or powdered sweetener

½ tsp fish sauce

Toppings

4 handfuls of beansprouts

3 spring onions, finely diced

4 tbsp chopped coriander

480g cooked chicken or beef, shredded or sliced

2 limes

4 tsp hoisin sauce

4 tsp sriracha

In a frying pan, fry the onion halves on a high heat for 1–2 minutes or until nicely charred.

Add the remaining base ingredients to a large pan along with the charred onion halves and gently simmer for 15–20 minutes, then remove the ginger, star anise and onion.

Add the noodles and cook for a further few minutes or until cooked, then divide the stock and noodles between 4 bowls. Add a handful of beansprouts, spring onions, coriander, cooked chicken or beef, a squeeze of half a lime per bowl, then finish with 1 teaspoon of hoisin and sriracha for each serving.

Optional: Add 1 teaspoon of chilli oil per portion for added flavour and kick!

KCAL	CARBS	PROTEIN	FAT	
432	56g	38g	8g	❄

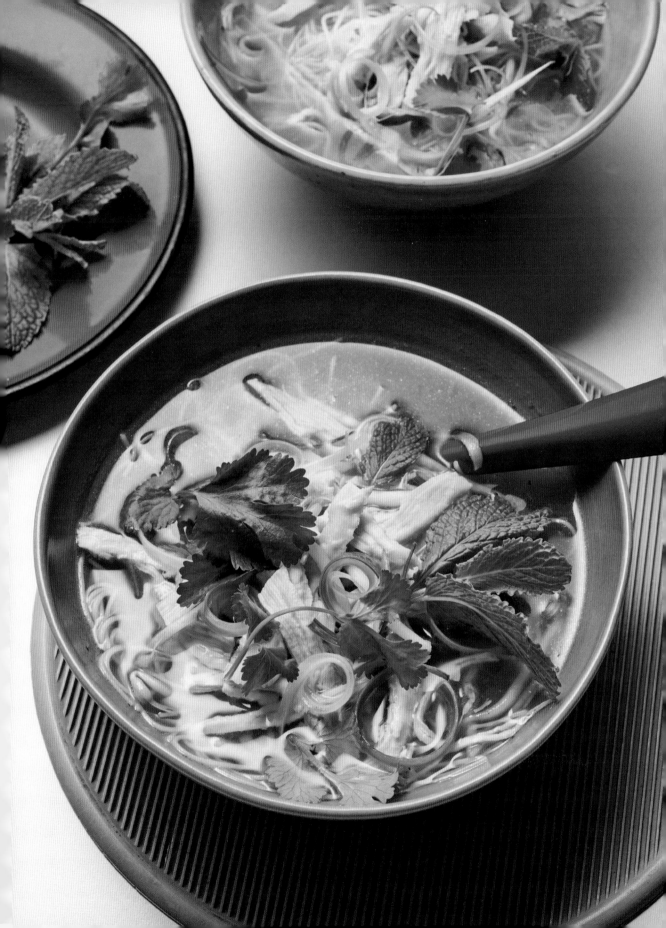

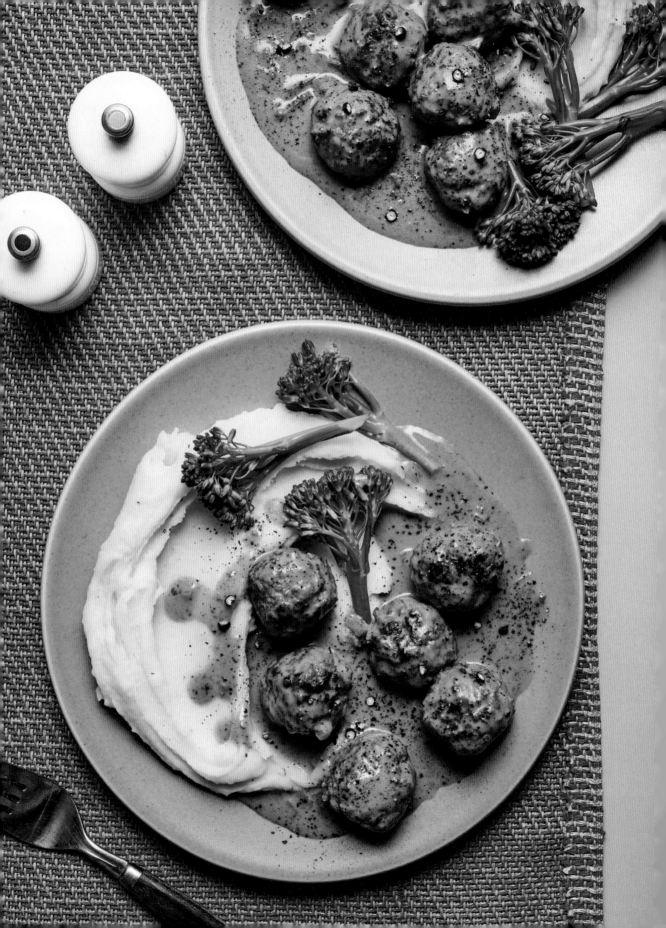

MINI MEATBALLS IN PEPPERCORN SAUCE

SERVES: 3 | **PREP**: 5–10 MINS | **COOK**: 12–14 MINS | GF + NF

One of my favourite steak sauces – a creamy peppercorn sauce. Instead of smothering it over steak, you're drenching mini beef meatballs in this mouth-watering peppery sauce.

500g lean beef mince
Low-calorie
  cooking spray
Salt and pepper
½ onion, finely diced
1 tbsp freshly ground
  black pepper
2 garlic cloves, minced
125ml beef stock
80ml reduced-fat
  crème fraîche
2 tsp cornflour mixed
  with 1–2 tbsp water
  to make a slurry

Side suggestions
Mashed potatoes
Broccoli

Make about 18 small meatballs from the beef mince, seasoning first with salt and pepper, and make sure they're compact. Spray a large pan with low-calorie cooking spray and cook the meatballs on a high heat for 3–4 minutes until they're nicely browned on all sides. Remove from the pan and set aside.

Spray the same pan with low-calorie cooking spray and fry the onion on a low heat for a couple of minutes to soften. Mix in the black pepper and garlic and fry for a further 1–2 minutes.

Pour in the beef stock, then mix in the crème fraîche. Add the meatballs back to the pan, making sure they're all coated in the sauce. Simmer on a low heat for 4–5 minutes or until the sauce starts to thicken. Add more ground pepper to your liking. Whisk in the cornflour if the sauce needs thickening.

KCAL	CARBS	PROTEIN	FAT	
314	13g	38g	14g	❄

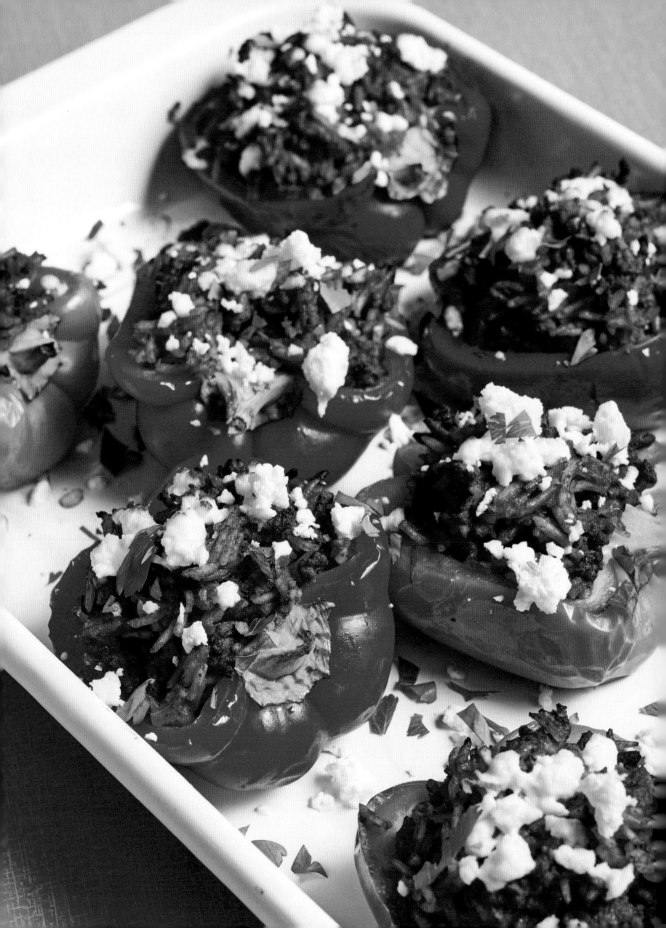

GREEK STUFFED PEPPERS WITH CRUMBLED FETA

SERVES: 4 | **PREP:** 5 MINS | **COOK:** 26–28 MINS | NF

A staple in Greece but made in half the time due to a few clever pre-cooking hacks. Each mouthful is exploding with Greek flavours and the crumbled feta just brings the dish to life.

4 large peppers (any colour)

Low-calorie cooking spray

1 red onion, finely diced

2 garlic cloves, minced

500g lean beef mince

½ tsp ground cinnamon

1 tsp dried oregano

Pinch of salt and pepper

450ml chicken stock

200g basmati rice

500g passata

100g feta, crumbled

2–3 tbsp finely chopped fresh parsley

Preheat the oven to 180°C.

Slice the peppers in half lengthways and remove the seeds and membrane. Place them cut-side down on a lined baking tray and spray with low-calorie cooking spray. Cook in the oven for 15 minutes.

Meanwhile, spray a large pan with low-calorie cooking spray and fry the onion for 2–3 minutes to soften, then add the garlic and beef mince. Fry for a couple of minutes, then add the cinnamon, oregano and salt and pepper and mix well.

Mix in the chicken stock, rice and passata, then simmer for 10 minutes or until all the stock has been absorbed and the rice is cooked.

Fill the peppers with the mince mixture and top with half of the feta. Oven-cook for 10–12 minutes, then garnish with the remaining crumbled feta and a sprinkle of parsley.

Air fryer method: Place the halved peppers cut-side down on a piece of foil in the air fryer and spray with low-calorie cooking spray. Air-fry at 180°C for 5–6 minutes to soften, then flip and fill, crumble over the feta and cook for a further 5–10 minutes.

KCAL	CARBS	PROTEIN	FAT		
490	59g	38g	12g		

BEEF KEEMA ALOO

SERVES: 4 | **PREP**: 5 MINS | **COOK**: 26–28 MINS | GF + DF + NF

Keema aloo is a curry that traditionally combines lamb mince with potatoes, peas and Indian spices. But instead, I'm using beef mince as it's cheaper and tastes amazing.

Low-calorie
  cooking spray

1 medium red or white
  onion, finely diced

2.5cm piece of fresh
  ginger, minced

2 garlic cloves, peeled
  and minced

500g lean beef mince

30g tomato purée

2 tbsp curry powder
  of your choice

1 large potato,
  peeled and cut into
  1.25cm cubes

400–500ml beef stock

200g frozen peas

2–3 tbsp finely
  chopped fresh
  coriander

Salt and pepper

Side suggestion
Basmati rice

**Swap: Change the
beef to lamb or
veggie mince.**

Spray a large pan with low-calorie cooking spray and fry the onion for a few minutes to soften, then add the ginger, garlic and beef mince.

Fry for 3–4 minutes, then add the tomato purée, curry powder and a good pinch of salt and pepper and mix well. Add the cubed potato and 400ml beef stock, mix well and simmer for 20 minutes or until the potato is tender, adding the extra 100ml stock if required. Add the frozen peas for the last few minutes of cooking.

Once cooked, sprinkle over the coriander and serve.

KCAL	CARBS	PROTEIN	FAT	
324	31g	34g	7g	

STICKY TERIYAKI GLAZED CHICKEN THIGHS

SERVES: 3 | **PREP**: 2 MINS | **COOK**: 10–12 MINS | DF + NF

Teriyaki sauce is a thing of beauty – it's sticky, sweet and salty and you can use it on just about any type of meat. This low-calorie homemade version is so, so easy to make, you won't go back to a shop-bought one. You can serve the teriyaki chicken with any type of rice or vegetables you fancy.

Low-calorie
   cooking spray
6 large skinless,
   boneless chicken
   thighs
Salt and pepper

Sauce
2 garlic cloves, minced
2.5cm piece of fresh
   ginger, peeeld
   and minced
1 tbsp soy sauce
1 tsp dark soy sauce
½ tsp white rice
   vinegar
1 tbsp honey
1 tbsp water

Side suggestions
Boiled green
   vegetables
Rice or noodles

**Swap: Use tamari
instead of soy
sauce to make
this gluten-free.**

Mix all the sauce ingredients together and set aside.

Spray a large frying pan with low-calorie cooking spray, season the chicken thighs with a good pinch of salt and pepper and fry on a medium–high heat for 4–5 minutes on each side.

Pour over the sauce and cook on a high heat for about a minute until it starts to bubble, making sure the chicken is coated on all sides. Once the sauce has reduced and becomes sticky, check that the chicken is cooked through, then serve.

Air fryer method: Marinate the chicken thighs in the sauce for 30 minutes, if you can, then air-fry at 200°C for 7 minutes. Coat the chicken in any leftover sauce and air-fry for a further 7 minutes, or until cooked. Pour any remaining sauce left in the air fryer over the chicken to serve.

KCAL	CARBS	PROTEIN	FAT		
329	6g	35g	17g		

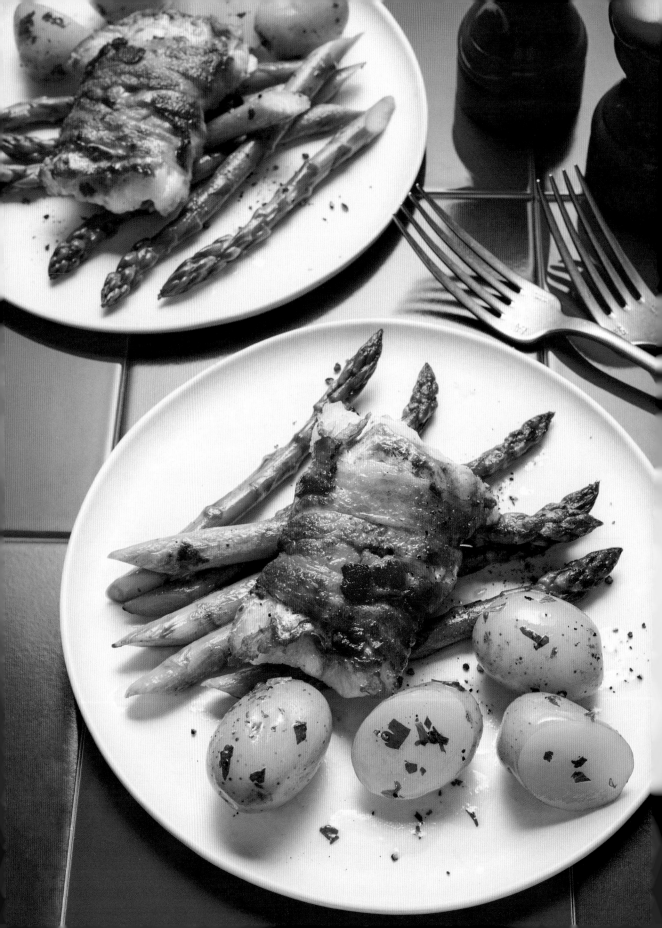

BACON-WRAPPED COD WITH CHEESY ASPARAGUS AND BUTTERY NEW POTATOES

SERVES: 2 | **PREP:** 5 MINS | **COOK:** 15 MINS | GF + NF

Want to change up your usual fish recipe? Add bacon to the mix, some cheesy asparagus and melt-in-the-mouth buttery new potatoes for the perfect fish dish.

350g new potatoes, halved

2 medium cod fillets

4 smoked bacon rashers

Low-calorie cooking spray

10 asparagus spears

40g reduced-fat Cheddar, grated

Salt and pepper

1 tbsp low-fat butter

1 tbsp fresh parsley, finely diced

Swap: You could use bacon medallions but they're super hard to wrap around the cod!

Boil the new potatoes in salted water for 15 minutes or until tender, then drain.

Meanwhile, season the cod fillets with salt and pepper, then wrap two bacon rashers around each fillet. Spray a frying pan with low-calorie cooking spray and add the cod and asparagus to the pan, seasoning the asparagus with salt and pepper. Cook the cod on a medium heat for 4 minutes on each side.

Remove the cod from the pan, then add the grated cheese over the asparagus. Place a lid over the pan to melt the cheese or just move it around in the pan until the cheese melts. At the same time, mix the butter and parsley with the potatoes and then serve with the cheesy asparagus and bacon-wrapped cod.

Air fryer method: Spray the bacon-wrapped cod with low-calorie cooking spray and air-fry at 190°C for 10–12 minutes or until the cod is cooked and the bacon is crispy. Flip halfway.

KCAL	CARBS	PROTEIN	FAT		
419	29g	45g	14g		

MOZZARELLA-STUFFED SAUSAGE AND BEEF MEATBALLS

SERVES: 4 | **PREP:** 5–10 MINS | **COOK:** 13–19 MINS | GF + NF

I'm a huge fan of any sort of meatballs, so for this recipe I fancied stuffing them with mozzarella and using a combo of sausage and beef mince for extra juiciness and flavour.

240g reduced-fat mozzarella ball

500g lean beef mince

8 reduced-fat pork sausages, skin removed

Low-calorie cooking spray

Salt and pepper

Grated Parmesan, to serve (optional)

Marinara sauce

500g passata

400g tin chopped tomatoes

1½ tsp dried oregano

1 tsp granulated or powdered sweetener

6–8 fresh basil leaves, torn

Side suggestion

Spaghetti, tagliatelle or any pasta

Dice the mozzarella ball into 20 small pieces and set aside.

Mix together the beef mince and pork sausages, season with a good pinch of salt and pepper, then roll into 20 balls. Push a piece of mozzarella into the centre of each ball, making sure the meat encloses the mozzarella tightly.

Spray a large frying pan with low-calorie cooking spray and cook the meatballs on a high heat for 3–4 minutes until browned on all sides. Add all the marinara sauce ingredients, including a good pinch of salt and pepper, carefully mix well and simmer for 10–15 minutes until the sauce has reduced.

Optional: Add grated Parmesan when serving.

KCAL	CARBS	PROTEIN	FAT	
444	16g	53g	19g	❄

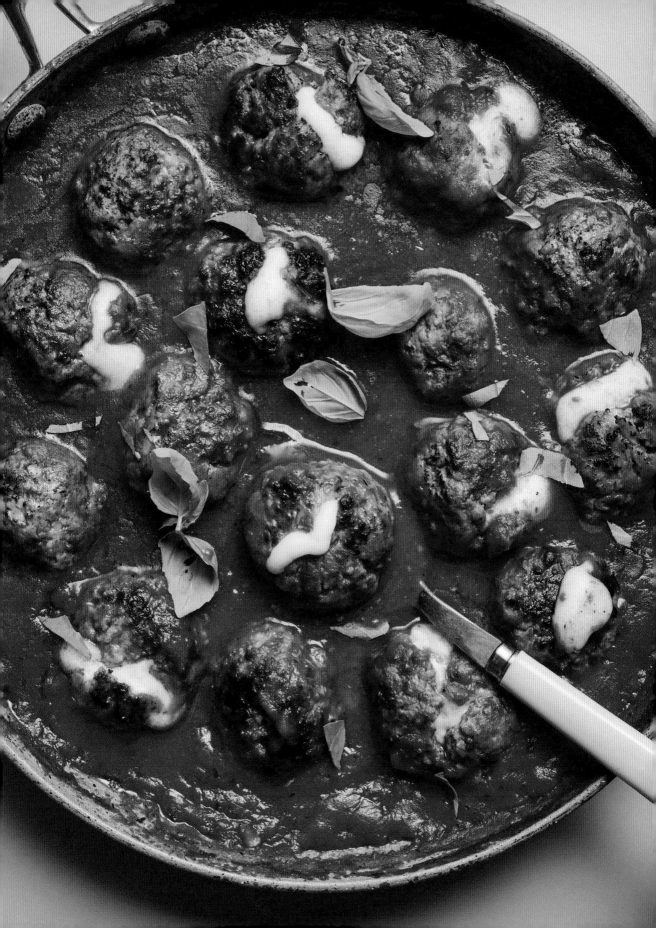

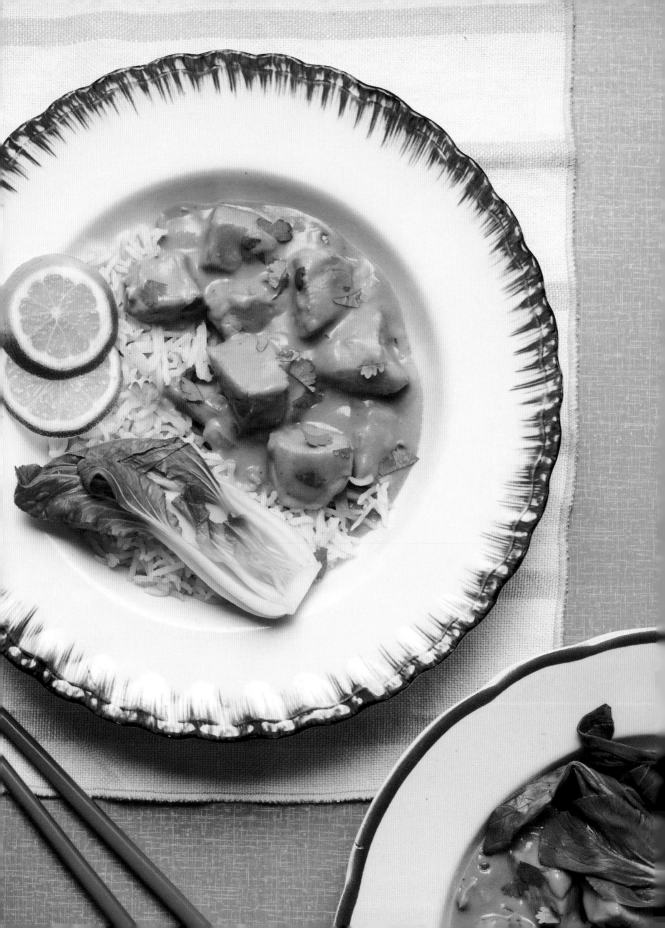

PEANUT BUTTER CHICKEN

SERVES: 2 | **PREP**: 2 MINS | **COOK**: 8–10 MINS | DF

Anything in a satay-style sauce and I'm here for it! It coats the chicken pieces wonderfully and I always make double so I can have some the next day too.

Low-calorie cooking spray

½ medium onion, finely diced

2 chicken breasts, diced

1 tsp soy sauce

2.5cm piece of fresh ginger, peeled and minced

1 garlic clove, minced

200ml chicken stock

2 tbsp smooth peanut butter

1 tsp granulated or powdered sweetener

2 tbsp finely chopped fresh coriander, to serve

A dollop of thick Greek yogurt or coconut milk (optional)

Side suggestions

Steamed green vegetables

Rice

Swap: Use tamari rather than soy sauce to make this gluten-free.

Spray a frying pan with low-calorie cooking spray and fry the onion for 2–3 minutes until softened.

Add the chicken and the soy sauce and make sure everything is coated well and fry for a further 5–6 minutes, adding the ginger and garlic for the last minute. Mix in the stock, peanut butter and sweetener and cook on a high heat for about a minute or until the sauce has thickened.

Sprinkle with the fresh coriander to serve.

Optional: If you fancy it super creamy, stir through a dollop of thick Greek yogurt or a splash of coconut milk before garnishing with the coriander.

KCAL	CARBS	PROTEIN	FAT
295	10g	45g	8g

MEDITERRANEAN FISH TRAYBAKE

SERVES: 4 | **PREP**: 5 MINS | **COOK**: 25–30 MINS | GF + DF + NF

Think of all the flavours of the Mediterranean in a fish traybake. It's one of those dishes that you just throw in the oven, and it comes out beautifully.

4 cod fillets
1 red pepper, diced
1 red onion, diced
250g cherry tomatoes
100g pitted
    Kalamata olives
1 lemon, halved
1 tbsp olive oil
1 tsp paprika
1 tsp dried oregano
Salt and pepper

Side suggestions
New potatoes or
    boiled rice mixed
    with coriander

Preheat the oven to 180°C.

Place the fish, vegetables and lemon halves in a large ovenproof dish and add the oil, paprika, oregano and some salt and pepper. Mix everything well and sit the fish on top of the other ingredients.

Oven-cook for 25–30 minutes or until the cod is cooked.

KCAL	CARBS	PROTEIN	FAT
217	8g	20g	11g

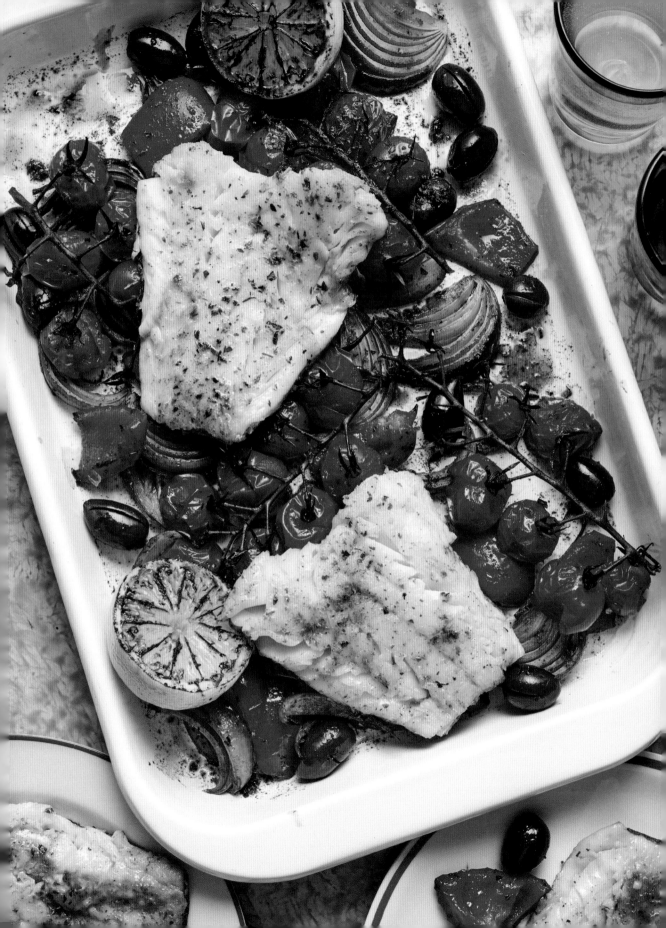

MIXED BEAN CHILLI WITH CRISPY CHEESE CROUTONS

SERVES: 3 | **PREP**: 5 MINS | **COOK**: 15–20 MINS | V + NF

One of the best vegetarian dishes I've ever made, especially with the crispy cheese croutons, which I could just eat a mountain of without a second thought. And the best part? It has 6 of your 5-a-day!

Low-calorie
  cooking spray
1 red onion,
  finely diced
1 green chilli,
  finely diced
3 garlic cloves, minced
½ tsp ground cumin
1 tsp smoked paprika
1 tsp mixed herbs
2 x 400g tins chopped
  tomatoes
250g vegetable stock
2 x 400g tinned
  mixed beans in
  water, drained
A handful of fresh
  coriander, finely
  chopped, to serve

Cheesy croutons
2 ciabatta rolls, cut
  into croutons
40g reduced-fat
  Cheddar, grated

Swap: Can't find the mixed beans? Grab a tin each of black beans, kidney beans, cannellini beans or chickpeas and take some from each tin.

Spray a large pan with low-calorie cooking spray and fry the onion and green chilli for a few minutes to soften, then add the garlic, spices and herbs. Mix well and fry for a further 1–2 minutes to release the aromas.

Mix in the remaining ingredients (apart from the coriander) and simmer for 15–18 minutes or until the liquid has reduced.

Spray a large frying pan with plenty of low-calorie cooking spray (or use a dash of olive oil) and fry the croutons on a high heat for a few minutes to brown.

Scatter over the grated cheese and keep flipping the croutons for 30 seconds until they are coated in the cheese and the cheese goes crispy. (They'll probably stick together, so use a spatula to break them apart.)

Serve each bowl of chilli with a sprinkle of coriander and a handful of croutons.

KCAL	CARBS	PROTEIN	FAT	
374	53g	22g	6g	

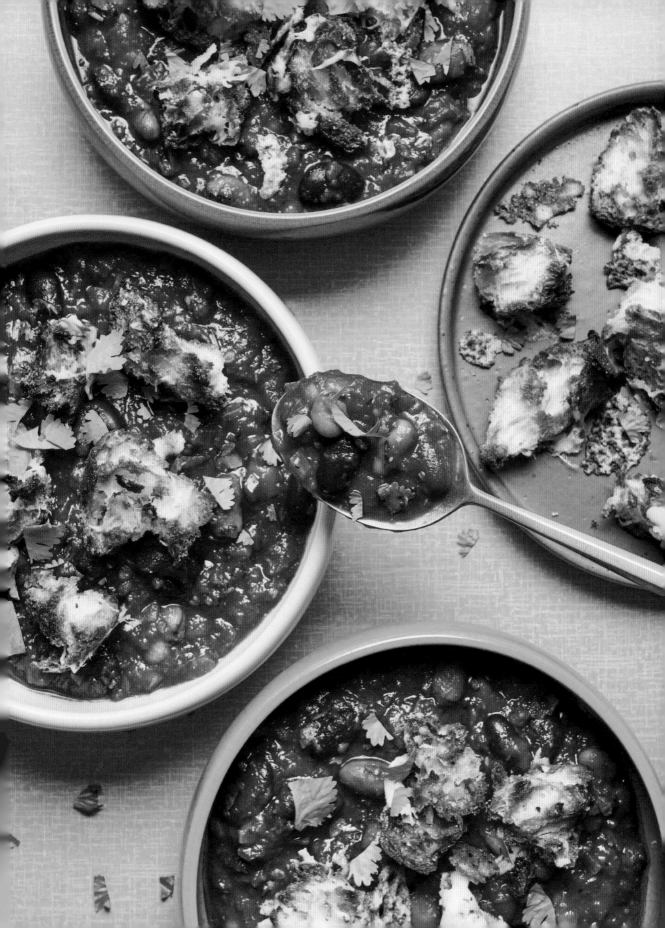

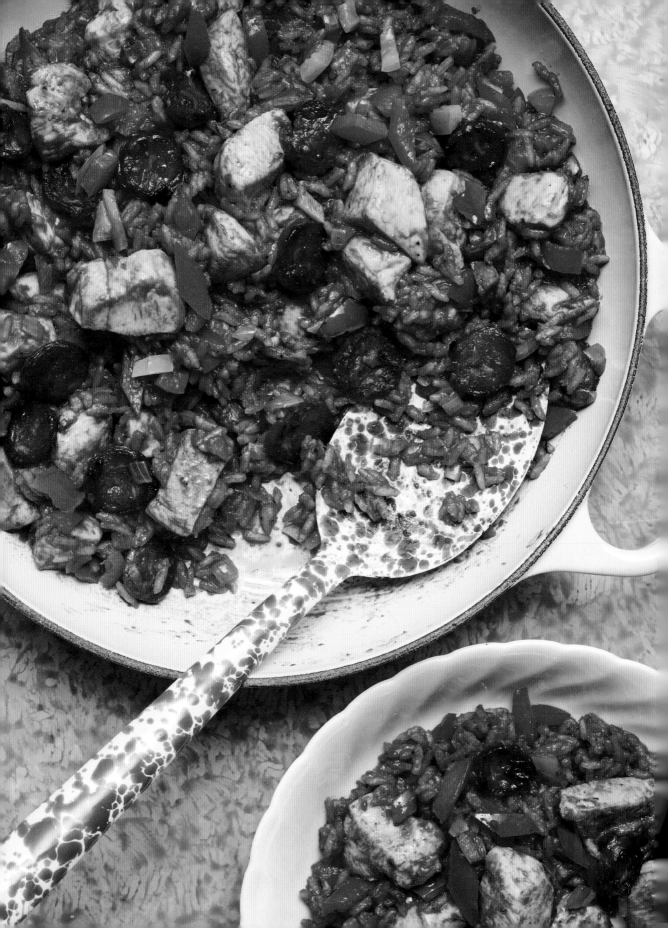

CHICKEN AND CHORIZO JAMBALAYA

SERVES: 4 | **PREP:** 5 MINS | **COOK:** 20–25 MINS | DF + NF

Jambalaya is an American savoury rice and meat dish. It's so flavoursome and easy to make and is perfect for any veg that need using up.

Low-calorie
  cooking spray
1 onion, finely diced
1 red pepper,
  finely diced
1 green pepper,
  finely diced
70g chorizo, sliced
3 chicken breasts,
  diced
500g passata
1 tbsp tomato purée
550ml chicken stock
200g long-grain rice
1 tbsp Cajun seasoning
2 tsp mixed herbs
Pinch of black pepper

Spray a large pan with low-calorie cooking spray and fry the onion for a few minutes to soften. Then add the peppers, chorizo and chicken and fry for a further 3–4 minutes until the chicken has browned.

Add the remaining ingredients, stir well and simmer for 18–20 minutes, stirring occasionally to prevent it from sticking, until all the stock has evaporated.

KCAL	CARBS	PROTEIN	FAT	❄
457	53g	40g	10g	

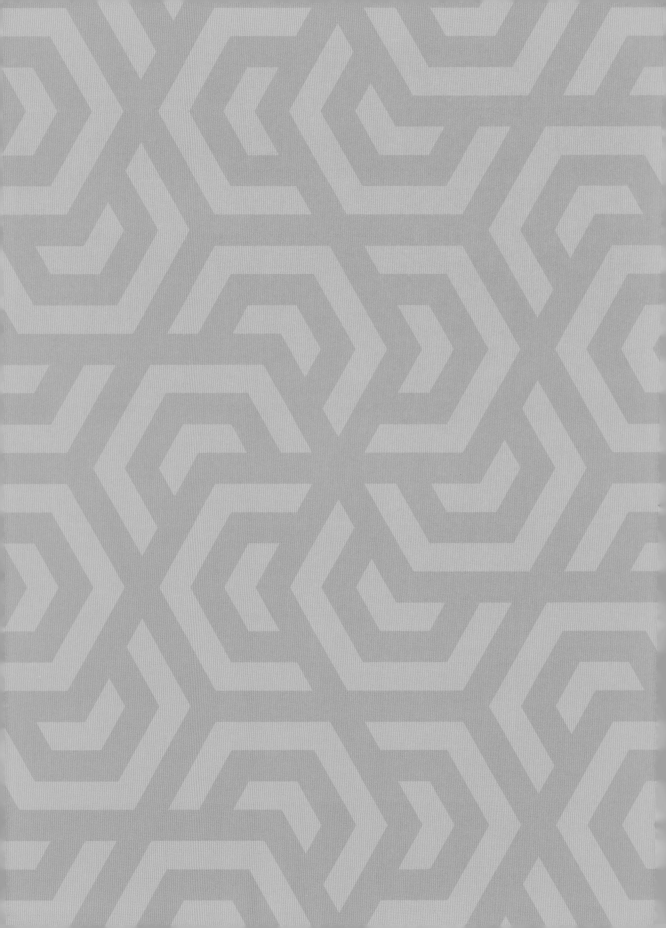

MEAL PREP WARRIORS

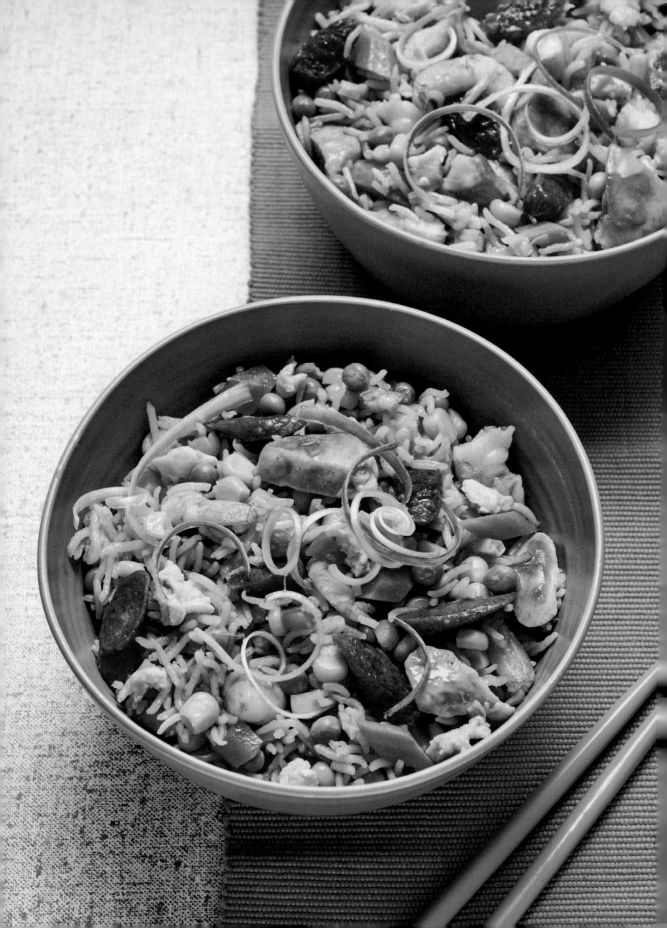

HOUSE SPECIAL
FRIED RICE

SERVES: 4 | **PREP:** 5 MINS | **COOK:** 10–12 MINS | DF + NF

Sometimes I just can't decide what my favourite fried rice is, so why not have the best of all worlds? This house special fried rice has chicken, salami and prawns, with a sauce that will delight your taste buds.

Low-calorie
  cooking spray
2 chicken breasts,
  sliced
45g salami sticks,
  sliced
300g frozen mixed
  vegetables
300g cooked king
  prawns, diced
5 eggs, beaten
200g cooked rice
1 tbsp soy sauce
½ tsp granulated
  or powdered
  sweetener (optional)
2 tbsp oyster sauce
Salt and pepper
Sliced spring onions,
  to serve (optional)

**Swap: Use tamari
instead of soy
sauce to make
this gluten-free.**

TIP: *If you have
any cooked
chicken left over,
from a roast for
example, then just
use that instead.*

Spray a large frying pan with low-calorie cooking spray and fry the chicken and salami on a medium–high heat for 5–6 minutes, then add the frozen veg and a dash of water. Fry for a further few minutes.

Add the king prawns and mix well, then move everything to one side of the pan, spray the other side with low-calorie cooking spray, add the eggs and scramble.

Once the eggs are cooked, mix in the cooked rice, then mix all the ingredients in the pan together. Season with the soy and oyster sauce making sure everything is coated evenly.

Optional: Add ½ teaspoon of sweetener when adding the soy sauce and serve with sliced spring onions.

KCAL	CARBS	PROTEIN	FAT	
442	35g	46g	13g	❄

SHREDDED HOISIN CHICKEN WRAPS

SERVES: 4 | **PREP:** 5 MINS | **COOK:** 6–8 MINS | DF + NF

Hoisin duck wraps from the Chinese takeaway are something I could eat every day, but they are fatty and not exactly low-calorie. So, I've made a healthy version by replacing the duck with chicken and they're as moreish as can be.

4 spring onions

1 cucumber

6 tbsp hoisin sauce

2 tsp soy sauce

4 chicken breasts

Low-calorie cooking spray

½ iceberg lettuce, sliced

8 mini tortilla wraps

Salt and pepper

Slice the spring onions and cucumber lengthways into thin strips resembling matchsticks and set aside.

For the sauce, mix 4 tablespoons of the hoisin sauce and the soy sauce with 2 tablespoons of water in a small bowl and set aside.

Butterfly the chicken breasts, then slice all the way through, so you've got two flat pieces per chicken breast. Season with salt and pepper. Spray a pan with low-calorie cooking spray and cook the chicken for 5–6 minutes or until cooked through. Remove from the pan and shred using two forks.

Place the shredded chicken back in the pan along with the sauce you made earlier and cook on a high heat for 1–2 minutes, making sure the chicken is well coated.

Warm the wraps in the microwave on high for 20–30 seconds, then spread the remaining hoisin sauce over the wraps evenly. Add the sliced lettuce, cucumber and spring onions to the wraps, then top with the chicken and roll up.

Air fryer method: Place the seasoned chicken in the air fryer, spray with low-calorie cooking spray and air-fry at 200°C for 10–12 minutes or until cooked through. Shred, then place the shredded chicken in a bowl and coat in the sauce. Wrap in foil and return to the air fryer for 2–3 minutes.

KCAL	CARBS	PROTEIN	FAT
445	50g	47g	6g

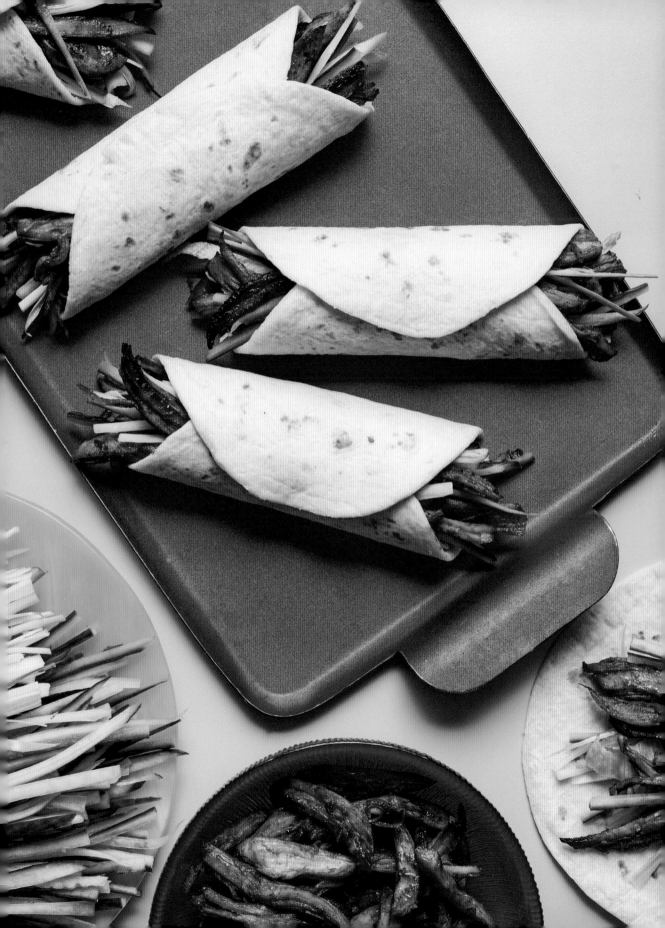

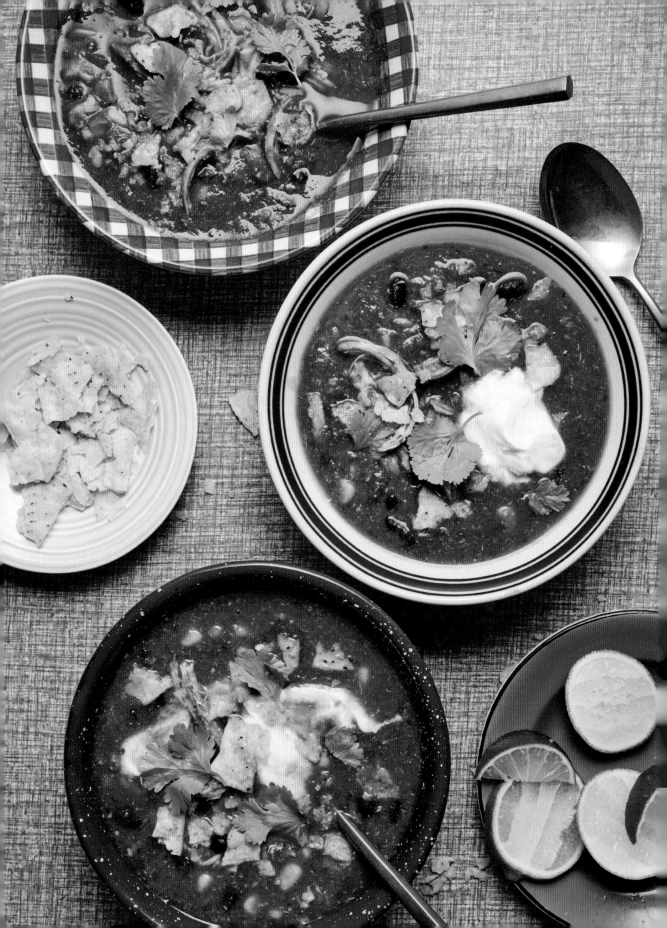

MEXICAN CHICKEN TORTILLA SOUP

SERVES: 4 | **PREP:** 5 MINS | **COOK:** 18–20 MINS | DF + NF

Do not be put off by the list of ingredients here – this is soup like you've never had it before. You'll probably have most of the ingredients to bring this Mexican soup to life at home already and the cherry on the cake is that it's topped off with tortilla chips.

Low-calorie
  cooking spray

1 medium onion,
  finely diced

3 garlic cloves, minced

40g jalapeños,
  finely diced

1 tsp paprika

1 tsp ground cumin

2 tsp chilli powder
  of your choice

400g tin chopped
  tomatoes

800ml chicken stock

200g tinned sweetcorn

3 tbsp finely chopped
  fresh coriander

400g tin black beans,
  drained and rinsed

3 chicken breasts

40g tortilla chips

1 lime, quartered

Salt and pepper

Soured cream or light
  crème fraîche, to
  serve (optional)

Spray a large, lidded pan with plenty of low-calorie cooking spray and fry the onion for 2–3 minutes to soften. Add the minced garlic, diced jalapeños and all the spices, along with a pinch of salt and pepper.

Fry for a further minute, then add the chopped tomatoes, chicken stock, sweetcorn, 2 tablespoons of coriander and the black beans. Mix well, then add the chicken breasts.

Pop on the lid and simmer for 15 minutes or until the chicken is cooked through. Remove the chicken from the soup and use two forks to shred it, then return it to the soup.

Add two ladles of the soup and 20g tortilla chips to a blender, blend, then add back into the soup, mixing well. Squeeze over a quarter of lime per portion and scatter over the remaining coriander. Crush up the remaining tortilla chips to sprinkle over the top.

Optional: Add a dollop of soured cream or light crème fraîche when serving.

KCAL	CARBS	PROTEIN	FAT
334	29g	39g	6g

CORONATION CHICKEN POTATO SALAD

SERVES: 4 | **PREP:** 5 MINS | **COOK:** 15 MINS | DF + NF

Two recipes combined into one – potato salad in a creamy, curried sauce with chicken pieces. This is an addictive dish.

700g new potatoes, halved

4 chicken breasts, diced into roughly 2cm chunks

Low-calorie cooking spray

2 handfuls of iceberg lettuce, sliced

Salt and pepper

Fresh coriander, chopped, to serve (optional)

Sultanas (optional)

Dressing

4 tbsp light mayonnaise

4 tbsp 0% fat Greek yogurt

1½ tbsp curry powder of your choice

1 tbsp mango chutney

3 spring onions, sliced

1 tsp lemon juice

Boil the new potatoes in salted water for 15 minutes or until tender, then drain and leave to cool.

Meanwhile, mix all the dressing ingredients together and set aside in the fridge.

Season the chicken breasts with a good pinch of salt and pepper and fry in a large frying pan with low-calorie cooking spray for 6–7 minutes or until cooked through. Set aside and leave to cool.

Add the chicken and new potatoes to a large bowl and mix in the dressing, then add the iceberg lettuce and divide between 4 plates.

Optional: Add a sprinkle of fresh coriander and some sultanas to each plate for a fresh flavour boost.

KCAL	CARBS	PROTEIN	FAT	
364	36g	50g	3g	

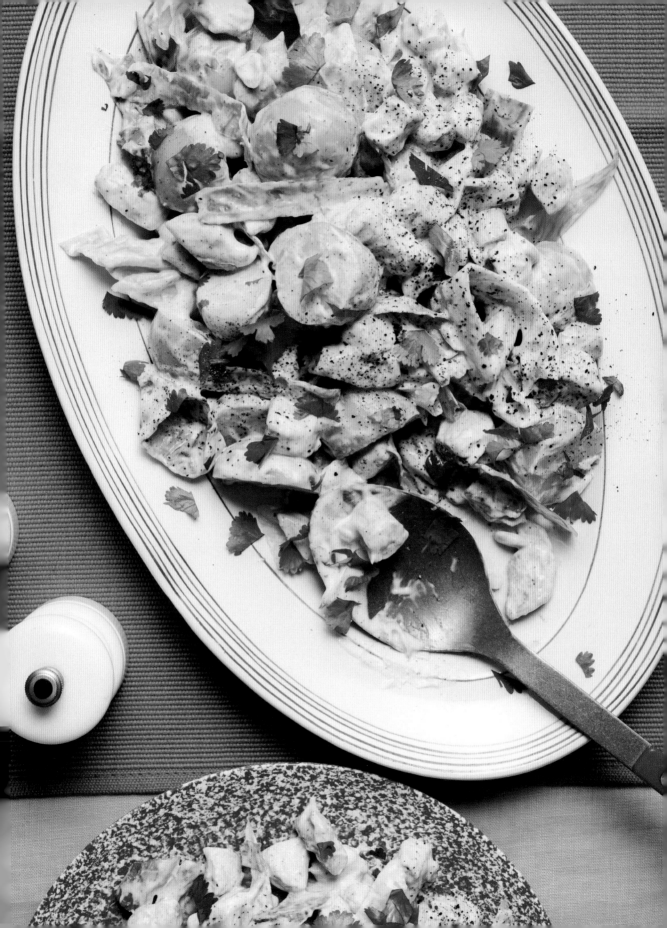

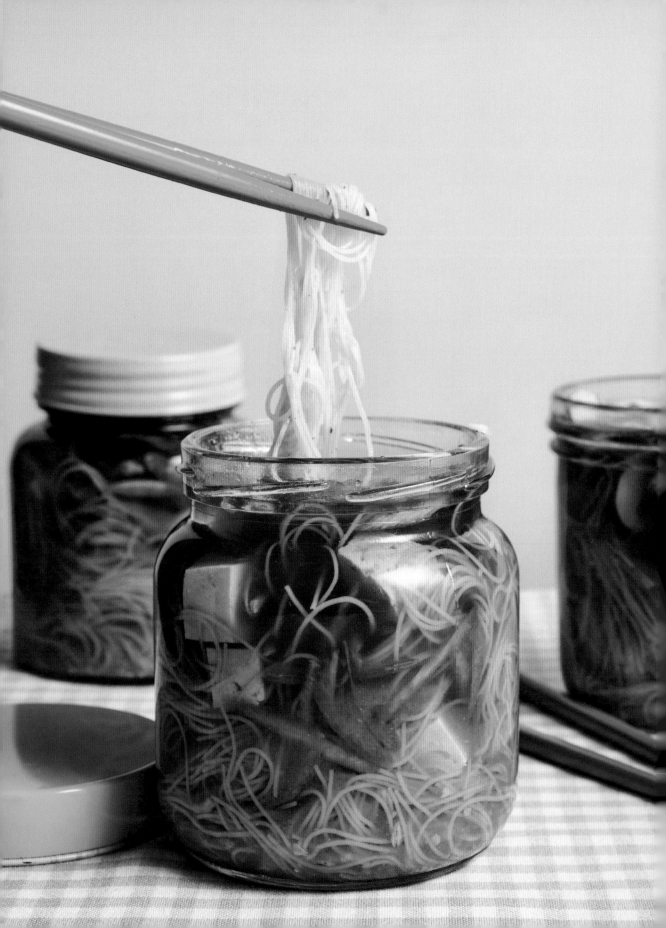

ON-THE-GO INSTANT NOODLES

SERVES: 4 | **PREP:** 5 MINS | **COOK:** 5–10 MINS | VE + DF + NF

This is a great recipe if you love noodles and need something to take with you on-the-go. With a tiny bit of prep, you can just fill these with boiling water, and you've got yourself a tasty, balanced meal.

4 nests of instant rice vermicelli noodles (225g)

2 carrots, grated

100g mangetout, thinly sliced lengthways

10 mushrooms, sliced

2 spring onions, sliced

320g cooked and marinated tofu pieces

Broth

4 vegetable or chicken stock cubes

4 heaped tsp miso paste

4 tsp soy sauce

4 tsp sesame oil

Swaps: Instead of tofu use shredded cooked chicken and swap soy sauce for tamari to make this gluten-free.

TIP: Any noodles would work with this, but some may take less time to cook than others.

Add all the broth ingredients to the bottom of 4 lidded glass jars or food containers, then place the noodles on top, then the veg and tofu.

When you're ready to eat, pour boiling water to cover all the ingredients, place the lid on and leave for 5–10 minutes, mixing well halfway. Enjoy!

KCAL	CARBS	PROTEIN	FAT	
374	52g	14g	12g	❄

SLOPPY JOE NACHOS

SERVES: 4 | PREP: 5 MINS | COOK: 16–18 MINS | NF

Sloppy Joes are basically loose meat sandwiches with beef mince and melty cheese in a rich tomato sauce which you take one bite of, and food gets everywhere. Think of this filling on top of a bed of nachos and, hey presto, you've got this recipe.

Low-calorie
cooking spray

1 medium onion,
finely diced

1 green pepper,
finely diced

500g lean beef mince

1 beef stock cube

120g reduced-fat
Cheddar, grated

3 tomatoes,
finely diced

80g tortilla chips

Seasoning

250g passata

3 tbsp reduced-sugar
tomato ketchup

1 tsp English mustard

A few dashes of
Worcestershire
sauce

1 beef stock cube

1 tsp granulated
or powdered
sweetener

Salt and pepper

To serve (optional)

Avocado, smashed

Jalapeños

Soured cream

Spray a large pan with low-calorie cooking spray and fry the onion and green pepper for a few minutes to soften. Add the beef mince and fry for a further 3–4 minutes.

Mix the beef stock cube with a few tablespoons of boiling water. Add to the beef with all the seasoning ingredients.

Fry on a medium heat for 5–10 minutes or until the sauce has reduced. Serve with everything on top of the tortilla chips and then add the grated Cheddar. Place under a hot grill until the cheese melts.

Optional: Some avocado, jalapeños and soured cream work wonders with this dish!

KCAL	CARBS	PROTEIN	FAT
360	24g	50g	12g

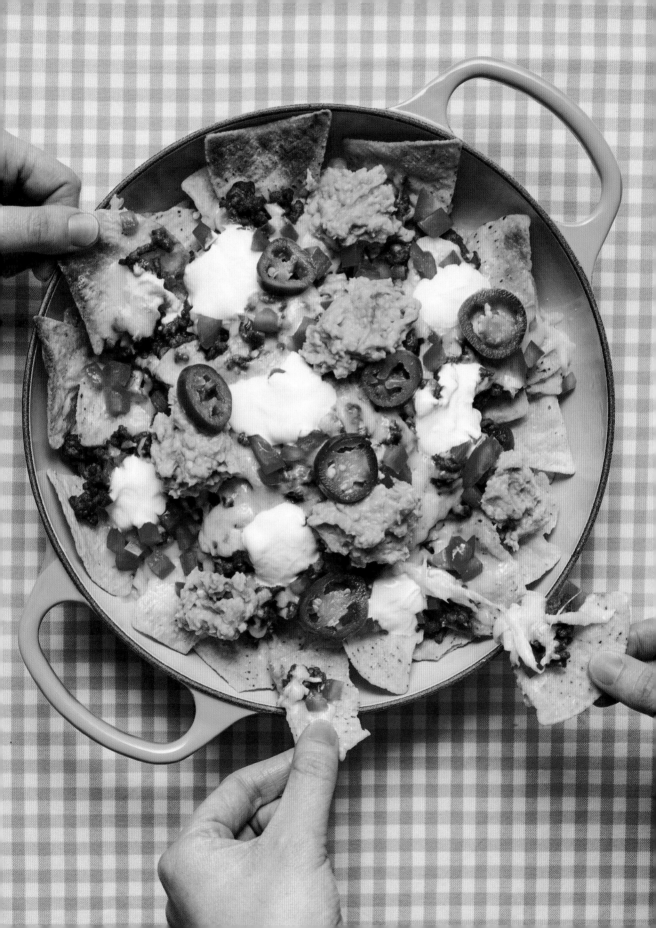

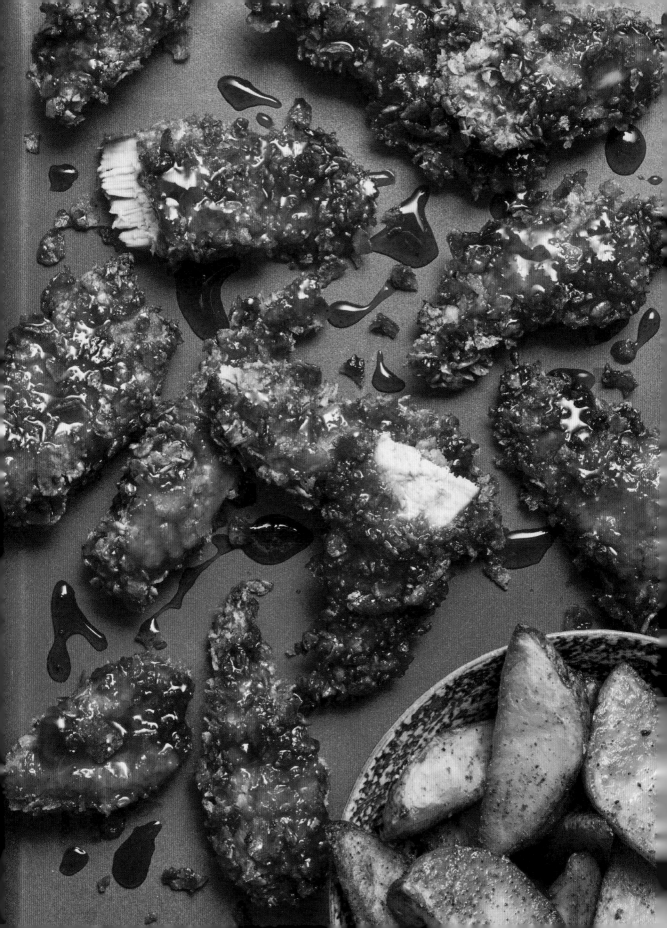

HONEY-BBQ CHICKEN TENDERS WITH POTATO WEDGES

SERVES: 4 | **PREP**: 5 MINS | **COOK**: 16–21 MINS | DF + NF

After sharing my first chicken tenders recipe on social media and it hitting over 7 million views, I knew it had to go into this book. I think it was the cornflake coating which makes the tenders super crispy that people were so amazed by!

Low-calorie
  cooking spray
4 chicken breasts
1 tbsp paprika
2 egg whites, beaten
110g cornflakes,
  crushed
Salt and pepper

Potato wedges
2 medium potatoes
2 tsp paprika
Salt and pepper

Glaze
5 tbsp BBQ sauce
3 tbsp honey
60ml water

Side suggestion
Mixed veg

Preheat the oven to 180°C.

Slice the potatoes into wedges, then season with salt, pepper and the paprika and place on a lined baking tray. Spray with plenty of low-calorie cooking spray.

Slice the chicken breasts into tenders, about 3–4 per fillet. Season with salt, pepper and the paprika, dip into the beaten egg whites, then coat in the cornflakes. Place on a lined baking tray, spray with low-calorie cooking spray and cook in the oven along with the wedges for 15–20 minutes or until cooked through. Turn the chicken and wedges halfway, spraying with more low-calorie cooking spray.

Pour the glaze ingredients into a pan and cook on a high heat for 30–60 seconds or until it starts to bubble, then pour over the chicken. Serve with the potato wedges.

Air fryer method: Place the chicken and wedges in the air fryer, spray with low-calorie cooking spray and air-fry at 200°C for 13–15 minutes for the chicken and 15–20 minutes for the wedges, turning halfway and spraying with more low-calorie cooking spray. (Cook in batches or cook the chicken and wedges separately if necessary.)

KCAL	CARBS	PROTEIN	FAT
436	56g	46g	3g

SPICY GOCHUJANG PEANUT NOODLES

SERVES: 4 | **PREP**: 2 MINS | **COOK**: 6–8 MINS | DF

Gochujang is an ingredient that I always have in my house as it makes a banging Korean sauce. But here I have mixed it with peanut butter for a spicy, salty, irresistible sauce that coats the noodles perfectly.

Low-calorie
  cooking spray
500g turkey mince
325g vegetable
  stir-fry mix
200g dried egg
  noodles, cooked
Salt and pepper
Sesame seeds and
  sliced spring onions,
  to serve (optional)

Sauce
4 tsp gochujang paste
2 tsp soy sauce
2 tbsp reduced-
  fat smooth
  peanut butter
1–2 tsp granulated
  or powdered
  sweetener
120ml water

Swaps: Use minced chicken, beef or even tofu and swap the soy sauce for tamari to make this gluten-free.

Mix all the sauce ingredients together and set aside.

Spray a large frying pan with low-calorie cooking spray and fry the turkey mince for 2–3 minutes, then add the stir-fry vegetables. Fry for a further 4–5 minutes or until the veg has softened, using more low-calorie cooking spray if needed.

Mix in the noodles, then the sauce and stir until everything is coated and serve.

Optional: Finish with a sprinkle of sesame seeds and sliced spring onions.

KCAL	CARBS	PROTEIN	FAT
431	43g	40g	10g

ROASTED CHIPOTLE CAULIFLOWER BOWL

SERVES: 4 | **PREP:** 5 MINS | **COOK:** 20–25 MINS | VE + DF + NF

Cauliflower is super versatile and holds on to flavour extremely well. Here I've coated it in spicy chipotle paste and made a beautiful, fresh sauce that effortlessly cools down the hotness of the chipotle. This is a dish not to miss if you love a range of flavours.

200g basmati rice

500g cauliflower, broken into small florets

4 tsp olive oil

1 tbsp chipotle paste

3 tomatoes, diced

1 medium avocado, diced

Dressing

A large handful of fresh coriander

2 tsp chipotle paste

2 garlic cloves

Juice of 1 lime

2 tbsp tahini

100ml water

Salt and pepper

Preheat the oven to 200°C.

Boil the rice as per the packet instructions and set aside.

In the meantime, coat the cauliflower florets in the olive oil and chipotle paste, then roast for 20–25 minutes or until tender and charred.

Meanwhile, add all the dressing ingredients to a blender, including a pinch of salt and pepper, and blend until smooth. Top the cooked rice with cauliflower, tomatoes and avocado. Pour over the dressing and serve.

Air fryer method: Air-fry the cauliflower at 200°C for 10–12 minutes, turning halfway.

KCAL	CARBS	PROTEIN	FAT		
389	52g	10g	16g		

DIRTY, CHEESY CAJUN RICE

SERVES: 4 | **PREP:** 5 MINS | **COOK:** 22–24 MINS | GF + NF

As the name suggests, this rice is seasoned to another level with Cajun seasoning and topped off with a handful of cheese to turn it into a cheesy taste sensation.

Low-calorie
  cooking spray
2 celery sticks,
  finely diced
1 large red pepper,
  finely diced
1 medium onion,
  finely diced
500g lean beef mince
2 garlic cloves, minced
4 tsp Cajun seasoning
20g tomato purée
200g basmati
  rice, washed
500g beef stock
100g reduced-fat
  Cheddar, grated
Salt and pepper
Sliced spring onions,
  to serve (optional)

Spray a large, lidded pan with plenty of low-calorie cooking spray and fry the finely diced vegetables for 3–4 minutes to soften.

Add the beef mince and garlic and fry for a further 3–4 minutes, then add the Cajun seasoning, tomato purée, a pinch of salt and a good pinch of pepper and mix well. Add the basmati rice and beef stock, mix again and stick the lid on.

Cook on a low heat for 12–14 minutes or until the stock has absorbed and the rice is cooked. Remove from the heat and top with the grated cheese, then stick the lid back on for 1–2 minutes to melt the cheese.

Optional: Scatter over some sliced spring onions to serve.

KCAL	CARBS	PROTEIN	FAT
470	52g	40g	13g

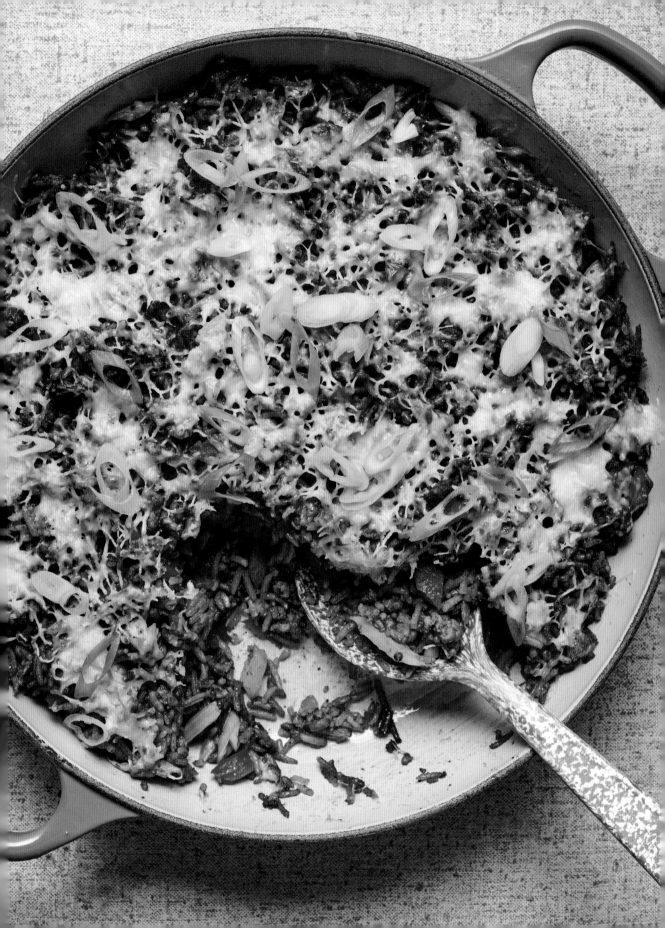

CHEESY BACON-STUFFED POTATO SKINS

SERVES: 4 | PREP: 5 MINS | COOK: 20–25 MINS | GF + NF

If you fancy a change from your usual jacket potato, make these delicious stuffed potato skins with bacon and creamy cheese. You can make them super quickly by using my microwave hack to speed up the cooking process.

4 medium potatoes

Low-calorie
    cooking spray

12 bacon medallions,
    cooked

90ml semi-
    skimmed milk

60g light soft cheese

2 spring onions,
    sliced

120g reduced-fat
    Cheddar, grated

Salt and pepper

Side suggestion
Side salad

Preheat the oven to 200°C.

Pierce the potatoes all over with a sharp knife and microwave on high for 5 minutes on each side.

Place the potatoes on a lined baking tray, spray with low-calorie cooking spray and top with a good pinch of salt. Bake in the oven for 10–15 minutes until crispy. Slice in half and leave to cool before scooping out the insides and placing in a large bowl.

Dice the bacon and mix with the remaining ingredients into the cooked potato, including a pinch of pepper, reserving half the Cheddar. Fill the potato skins with the filling, then pop the reserved Cheddar on top and return to the oven for a further 5–6 minutes. Sprinkle over the spring onions to serve.

Air fryer method: After microwaving, place the potatoes in the air fryer, spray with low-calorie cooking spray and top with salt. Air-fry at 200°C for 12 minutes. Fill, then air-fry for a further 5–6 minutes.

KCAL	CARBS	PROTEIN	FAT		
336	40g	35g	5g		

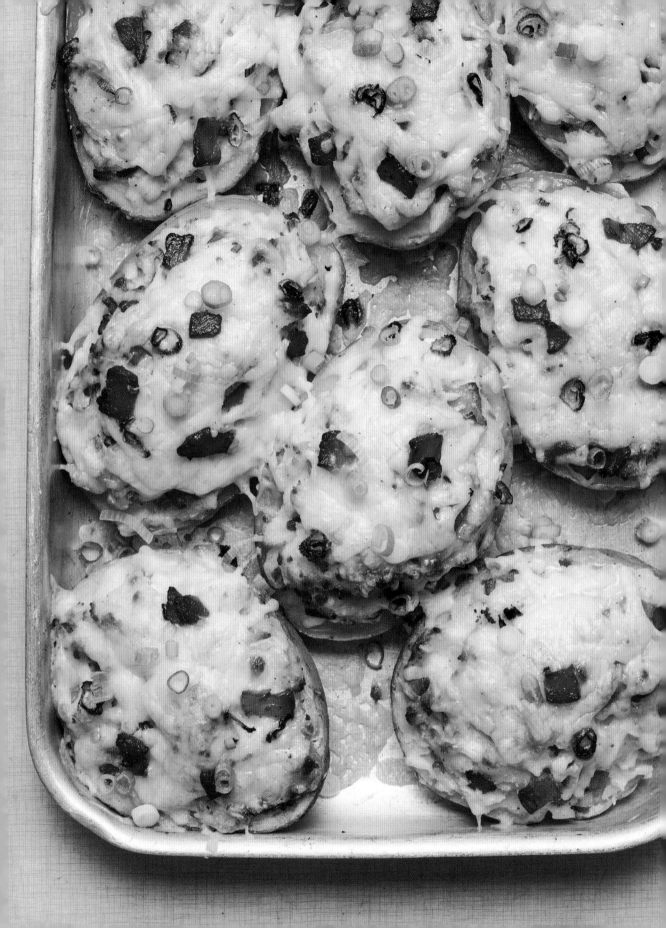

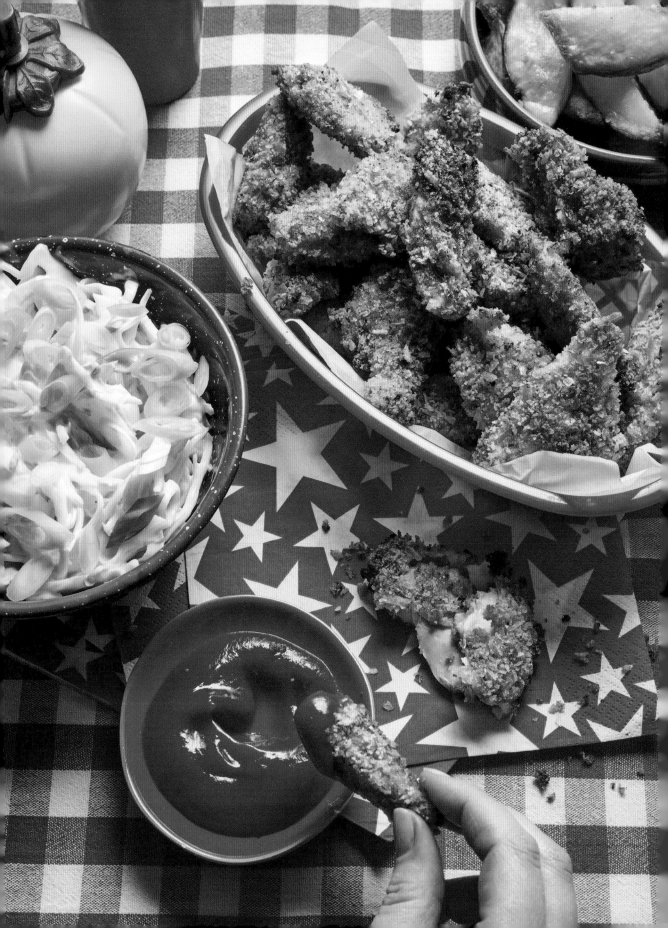

SOUTHERN NOT-SO-FRIED CHICKEN AND SLAW

SERVES: 4 | **PREP:** 5 MINS | **COOK:** 8–10 MINS

Healthy fried chicken – are you serious? The answer is yes, I am. I know it's not exactly fried, but it tastes very similar and teamed with the creamy slaw and some homemade potato wedges, your family will be asking you to make this on the regular.

6 medium skinless, boneless chicken thighs

2 eggs, beaten

70g dried breadcrumbs

Low-calorie cooking spray

Salt and pepper

Slaw

80g white cabbage, sliced

2 carrots, grated

2 spring onions, sliced

4 tbsp light mayonnaise

4 heaped tbsp low-fat natural yogurt

1 tsp English mustard

Squeeze of lemon juice

Southern fried chicken seasoning

2 tsp paprika

2 tsp onion granules

2 tsp garlic granules

1 tsp cayenne pepper

1 tsp dried oregano

Side suggestion

Homemade potato wedges (see page 131)

Preheat the oven to 180°C.

Mix all the slaw ingredients together and set aside in the fridge.

Slice the chicken thighs lengthways into 2.5cm strips, then season with salt and pepper. Mix the breadcrumbs with the southern fried chicken seasoning ingredients and a good pinch of salt and pepper, dip the chicken into the beaten eggs, then into the seasoned breadcrumbs.

Place the coated chicken on a lined baking tray and spray with low-calorie cooking spray. Cook in the oven for 15–20 minutes, turning halfway and spraying with more low-calorie cooking spray.

Serve the chicken with the slaw alongside.

Air fryer method: Spray the chicken with low-calorie cooking spray and air-fry at 200°C for 4–5 minutes, flip, then spray with more low-calorie cooking spray. Take the chicken out of the air fryer and leave to rest for 4 minutes before serving with the slaw.

Swaps: You can use panko breadcrumbs and chicken breast instead.

KCAL	CARBS	PROTEIN	FAT		
367	26g	31g	15g		

BLACKENED HADDOCK WITH BUTTERY SWEETCORN RICE

SERVES: 4 | **PREP:** 2 MINS | **COOK:** 6 MINS | GF + NF

A smoky, bold blackened seasoning with flaky tender haddock teamed up with a delicious buttery sweetcorn rice. A perfect match.

200g basmati rice
4 haddock fillets
Low-calorie cooking spray
200g tinned sweetcorn, drained
3 tbsp low-fat butter

Seasoning
5 tbsp light mayonnaise
1 tsp smoked paprika
1 tsp garlic granules
1 tsp onion granules
1 tsp dried parsley
Pinch of salt and pepper

Swap: Use cod or salmon if you don't fancy haddock.

Cook the rice according to the packet instructions and set aside.

Meanwhile, in a bowl mix the seasoning ingredients together and brush over the haddock fillets. Spray a large frying pan with low-calorie cooking spray and pan-fry the haddock for 3 minutes on each side, spraying with more low-calorie cooking spray when flipping so the fish doesn't stick to the pan. (Cook in batches if required to not overcrowd the pan.)

Mix the cooked rice with the sweetcorn and butter, then season with salt and pepper. Serve with the haddock fillets.

<u>**Air fryer method:**</u> Air-fry the seasoned haddock at 180°C for 8–10 minutes.

KCAL	CARBS	PROTEIN	FAT		
367	50g	28g	7g		

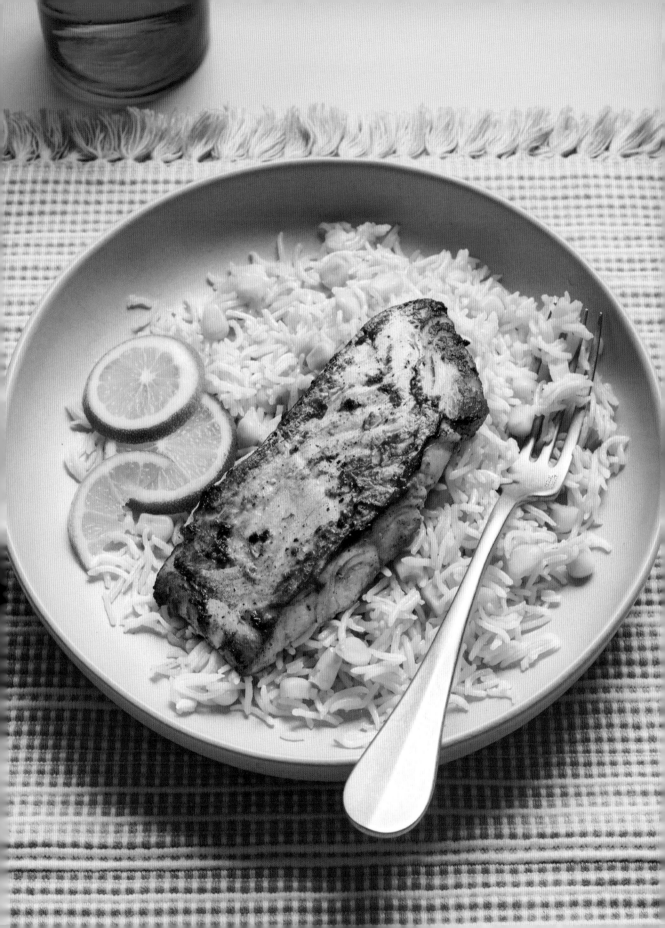

FAKEAWAYS

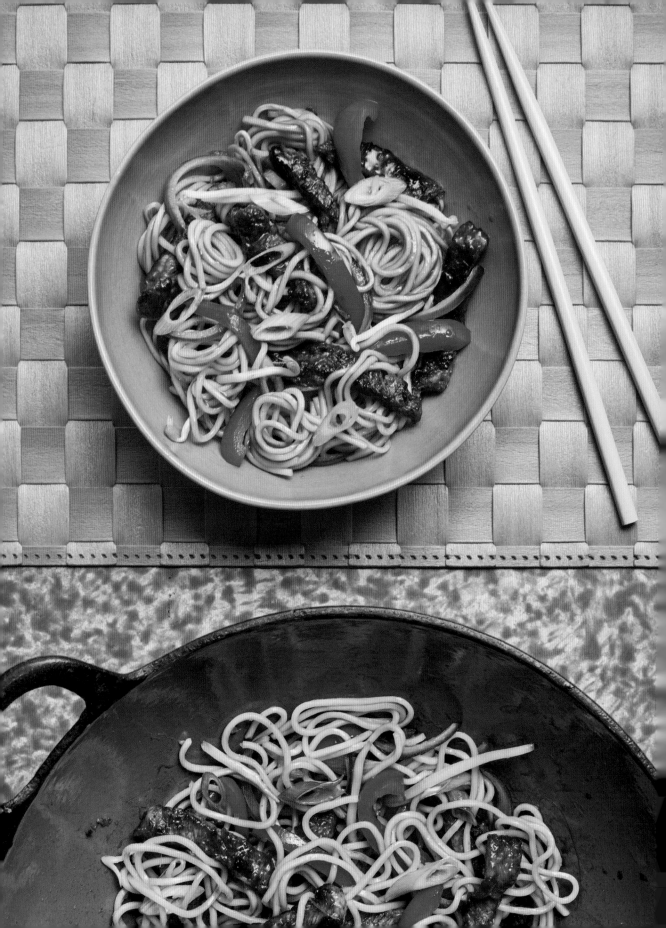

MONGOLIAN BEEF NOODLES

SERVES: 2 | **PREP**: 5 MINS | **COOK**: 8–10 MINS | DF + NF

Mongolian beef is thinly sliced beef in a super simple rich sauce made from soy sauce and brown sugar. I use a little trick to make the beef extra tender by using a secret ingredient: baking powder. It breaks down the beef, which helps to keep it tender and moist.

200g sirloin or ribeye steak, fat removed, sliced

1 tsp soy sauce

10g cornflour

¼ tsp baking powder

Low-calorie cooking spray

½ red onion, sliced

½ red pepper, sliced

1 garlic clove, minced

2.5cm piece of fresh ginger, peeled and minced

A handful of beansprouts

100g dried egg noodles, cooked

Sliced spring onions, to serve (optional)

Sauce

1 tbsp soy sauce

1 tbsp dark soy sauce

2 tbsp light brown soft sugar

2–3 tbsp water

TIP: *You can pretty much add in any veg you want to this dish!*

In a bowl, mix together all the sauce ingredients and set aside.

Marinate the steak slices in the soy sauce, cornflour and baking powder.

Spray a large frying pan with low-calorie cooking spray and fry the onion and red pepper for a few minutes to soften, then mix in the garlic, ginger and beansprouts. Fry for a further 1–2 minutes.

Remove the veg from the pan, spray with more low-calorie cooking spray and fry the steak on a high heat for 2–3 minutes. Remove, pour in the sauce, and cook on a high heat until the sauce starts to bubble.

As soon the sauce bubbles, add the cooked noodles, beef and veg, mixing well until everything is coated.

Optional: Add a sprinkle of sliced spring onions when serving.

KCAL	CARBS	PROTEIN	FAT	
439	64g	32g	6g	❄

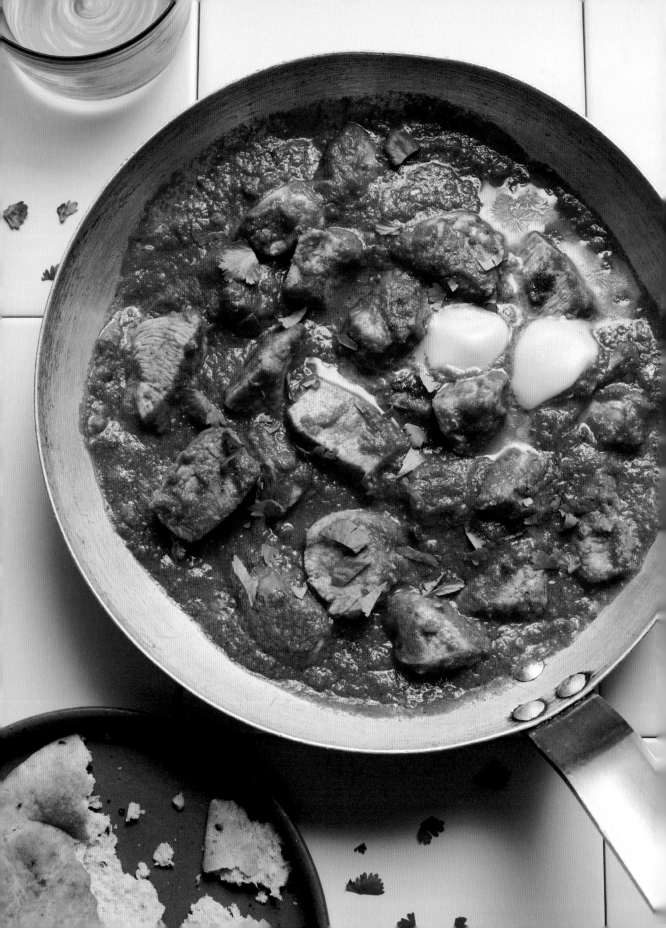

BUTTER CHICKEN

SERVES: 2 | **PREP**: 5 MINS (+30 MINS MARINATING) | **COOK**: 13–15 MINS | GF + NF

A creamy, obviously buttery, butter chicken that goes stupidly well with naan or flatbreads to dip into the sauce. I'll never get bored of this dish.

2 chicken breasts, diced

Low-calorie cooking spray

½ medium onion, finely diced

400g tin chopped tomatoes

60ml single cream

1 tbsp low-fat butter

A sprinkle of fresh coriander, to serve (optional)

Marinade

1 tsp olive oil

1 garlic clove, minced

2.5cm piece of fresh ginger, peeled and minced

1 tbsp garam masala

1 tsp ground turmeric

2 tsp paprika

½ tsp salt

5 heaped tbsp fat-free Greek yogurt

Squeeze of lemon juice

Side suggestions

Basmati rice

Naan

First, make the marinade. Mix the oil, garlic and ginger, half the spices, the salt, 4 heaped tablespoons of the yogurt and the lemon juice together in a bowl. Add the chicken pieces and stir to coat and if you have time, leave to marinate for 30 minutes.

Spray a pan with low-calorie cooking spray and cook the chicken on a medium heat for 6–7 minutes. Remove from the pan and set aside. In the same pan, fry the onion in more low-calorie cooking spray for a few minutes to soften, then add the remaining spices and fry for a further few minutes.

Transfer the onion to a blender and add the chopped tomatoes, the remaining 1 tablespoon of Greek yogurt and the cream and blend until smooth. Return the sauce to the pan along with the chicken and cook on a medium–high heat for 1–2 minutes.

Mix in the butter, sprinkle with coriander (if using) and serve.

KCAL	CARBS	PROTEIN	FAT
420	19g	56g	14g

CRISPY CHICKEN RICE BOX

SERVES: 2 | **PREP**: 5 MINS | **COOK**: 16–18 MINS | DF + NF

You may be able to guess where I got the inspiration for this recipe . . .
I use chilli tortilla chips for the chicken coating to make this taste just like the
real thing (I'm still shocked every time I taste it!), with homemade Mexican
rice and salad. You'll be saving a lot of money by making this at home!

30g chilli-flavoured
   tortilla chips (I
   like Doritos Chilli
   Heatwave)

2 chicken breasts

1 egg, beaten

Low-calorie
   cooking spray

2 handfuls of
   lettuce, sliced

1 tomato, finely diced

Garlic mayonnaise,
   to serve (optional)

Rice

100g frozen mixed veg

½ vegetable
   stock cube

50ml boiling water

A pinch of ground
   turmeric

200g cooked rice

Preheat the oven to 180°C.

Bash the tortilla chips into big crumbs in a freezer bag. Dip the
chicken into the beaten egg, then the tortilla crumbs. Place the
coated chicken on a lined baking tray, spray with low-calorie
cooking spray and cook in the oven for 16–18 minutes,
turning halfway.

For the rice, add the frozen veg to a pan, along with the
vegetable stock cube and water and simmer for a few minutes
until the veg has defrosted and most of the water has gone,
then mix in the turmeric and finally the cooked rice.

Slice the chicken and serve on top of the lettuce, tomatoes
and rice.

Optional: I love adding a drizzle of garlic mayonnaise to this.

Air fryer method: Spray the coated chicken with low-calorie
cooking spray and air-fry at 200°C for 10–15 minutes.

KCAL	CARBS	PROTEIN	FAT		
443	46g	48g	8g		

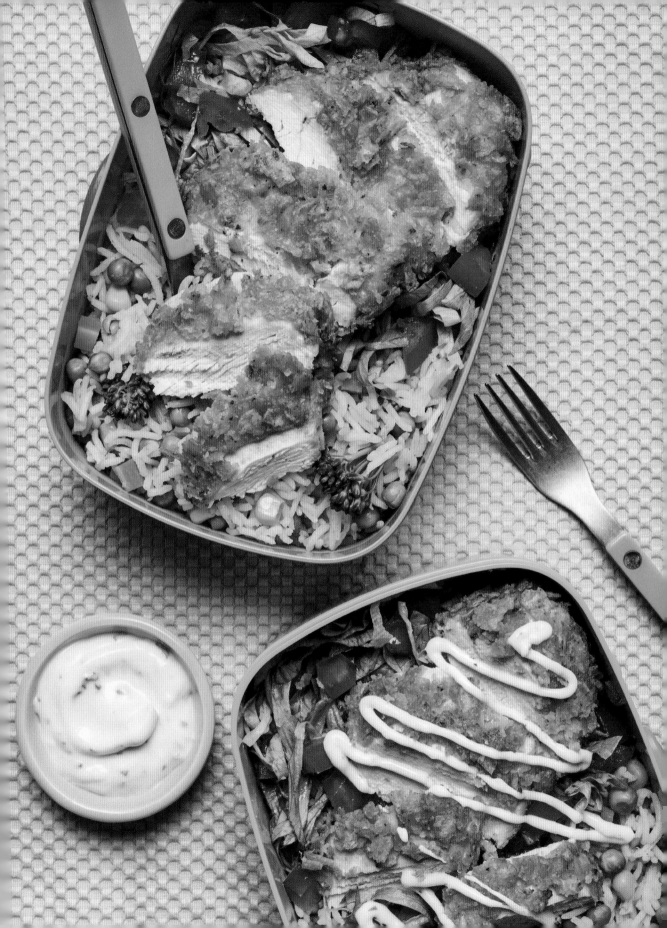

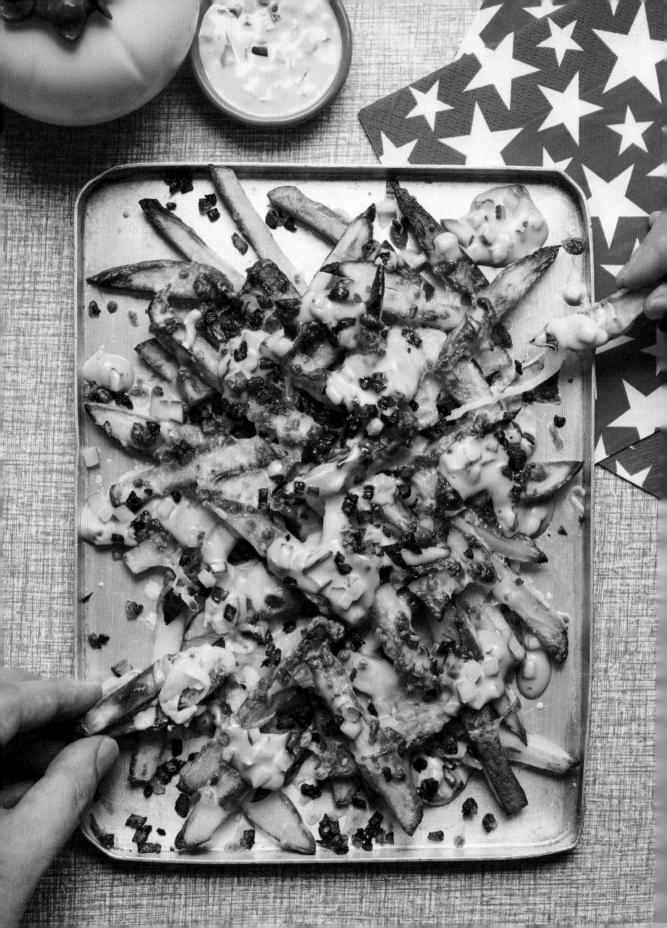

ANIMAL-STYLE FRIES

SERVES: 2 | **PREP**: 2 MINS | **COOK**: 15 MINS | NF

There's a fast-food chain in America that is well known for these one-of-a-kind, moreish fries – I haven't had fries like them. They're basically crispy fries drenched in burger sauce (I could drink the stuff), with crispy, caramelised onions. Perfect with a homemade burger or as a snack.

2 medium potatoes, sliced into fries

Low-calorie cooking spray

½ large onion, finely diced

1 tsp soft light brown sugar

40g shredded mozzarella

Salt

Sauce

6 tbsp light mayonnaise

3 tbsp reduced-sugar tomato ketchup

1 medium gherkin, finely diced (with a dash of juice)

1 tsp English mustard

> **TIP**: *You can fry the onions on a low heat for 20-25 minutes to caramelise them, but I just don't have the patience!*

Preheat the oven to 180°C.

Mix all the sauce ingredients together with a dash of gherkin juice and set aside in the fridge.

Place the fries on a lined baking tray and spray with plenty of low-calorie cooking spray, then season well with salt. Cook in the oven for 15 minutes, making sure to flip them halfway and spray again with more low-calorie cooking spray so that they crisp up nicely.

Meanwhile, spray a pan with low-calorie cooking spray and fry the onion on a medium heat for 10 minutes or until lovely and crispy. Sprinkle over the brown sugar for the last few minutes of cooking, stirring well.

To assemble – chips first, then mozzarella, put back in the oven, under the grill or in the microwave until melted, then drizzle over the homemade sauce and top with the crispy onions.

Air fryer method: Spray the fries with low-calorie cooking spray and air-fry at 200°C for 15 minutes, turning halfway and spraying more low-calorie cooking spray.

KCAL	CARBS	PROTEIN	FAT
302	53g	10g	6g

BANGING BEEF BURRITO

SERVES: 2 | **PREP:** 2 MINS | **COOK:** 8–10 MINS | GF + NF

A warm tortilla wrap filled with a number of juicy fillings including beef mince, kidney beans and Mexican rice. This is a lunchtime favourite you can throw together in less than 10 minutes!

250g lean beef mince

Low-calorie cooking spray

1 tbsp taco seasoning

2 heaped tbsp red kidney beans

2 tortilla wraps

40g reduced-fat Cheddar, grated

125g shop-bought Mexican rice, cooked

2 handfuls of iceberg lettuce, sliced

1 tomato, finely diced

Jalapeños (optional)

Soured cream (optional)

In a frying pan, fry the beef mince in low-calorie cooking spray for 3–4 minutes, then season with the taco seasoning. Add a dash of water and the kidney beans, then fry for a further few minutes.

To assemble, grab the wraps, then divide the beef mixture between them. Top with the cheese, rice, lettuce and tomato, plus a few jalapeños and a dollop of soured cream if you like. Roll up into burritos and fry on all sides in the same pan as before, sprayed with low-calorie cooking spray, for a few minutes to brown. Wrap in some foil for a real burrito experience and enjoy!

Optional: Add a few jalapeños and a dollop of soured cream before wrapping.

KCAL	CARBS	PROTEIN	FAT
471	51g	44g	9g

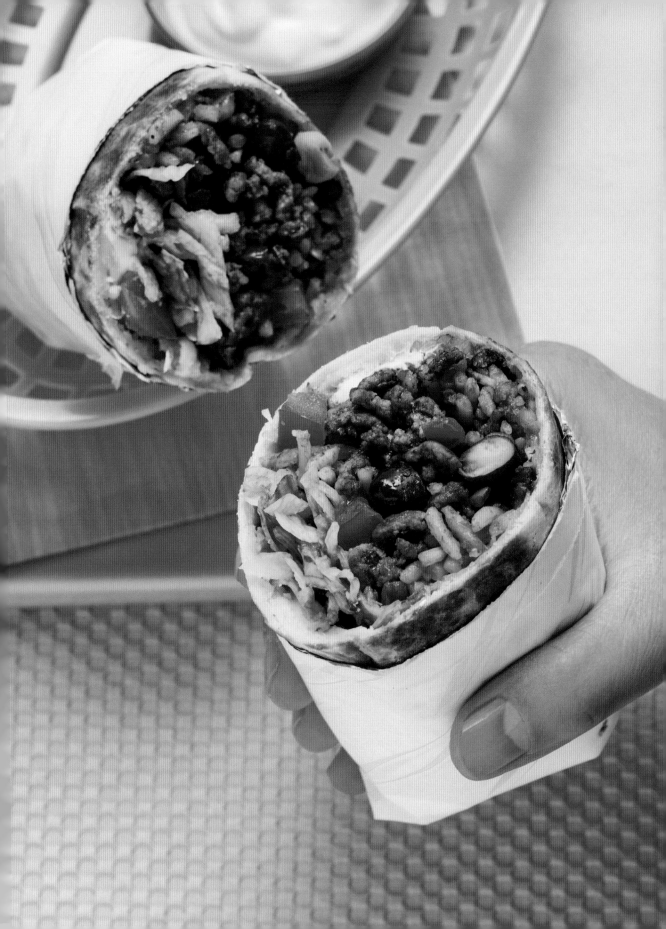

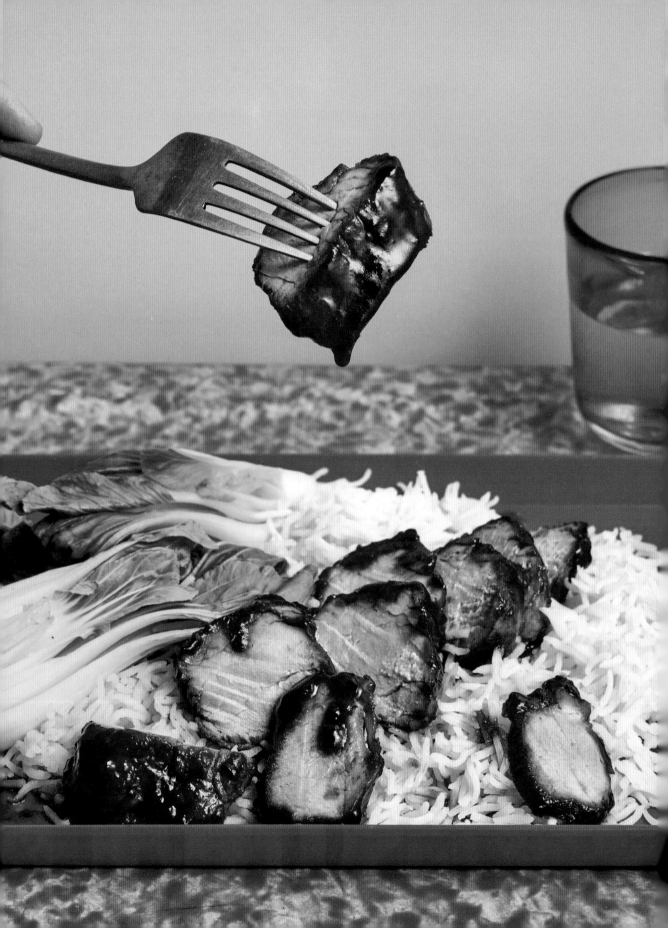

CHAR SIU PORK

SERVES: 3 | **PREP**: 2 MINS (+1 HOUR MARINATING | **COOK**: 14–16 MINS | DF + NF

Red-tinted pork is what I think of when I think of char siu pork. It's a Chinese BBQ pork flavoured with a wonderfully fragrant spice – Chinese five spice – and it's super easy to make at home.

480g lean pork
    tenderloin

1 tsp sesame oil

2 tbsp soy sauce

2 tbsp hoisin sauce

1 tbsp honey

2 garlic cloves, minced

1 tsp Chinese
    five spice

Red food colouring
    (optional)

Side suggestions

Pak choi

Rice

**Swap: Swap soy
sauce for tamari
to make this
gluten-free.**

Mix all the ingredients together and marinade the pork for at least 1 hour or overnight for the best results.

Grill the pork on high for 14–16 minutes, depending on the size, flipping halfway and basting with any spare marinade. Rest for 6–8 minutes, then slice and serve.

Optional: Mix in some red food colouring for that char siu pork colour.

Air fryer method: Air-fry at 200°C for 14–16 minutes, flipping halfway and basting with any spare marinade. Rest for 6–8 minutes before slicing.

KCAL	CARBS	PROTEIN	FAT		
317	14g	52g	5g		

CHICKEN PARMO

SERVES: 2 | **PREP**: 5 MINS | **COOK**: 15–18 MINS | NF

A staple up north, I first found out about this delicacy during a university night out on Teesside. A chicken escalope drenched with béchamel and topped with more cheese. But I've made a low-calorie version and it's just as indulgent.

2 chicken breasts
1 egg, beaten
40g panko breadcrumbs
Low-calorie cooking spray
40g reduced-fat Cheddar
Salt and pepper

Béchamel
1 tbsp low-fat butter
15g plain flour
130ml semi-skimmed milk
A pinch of nutmeg

Side suggestions
Homemade chips (see page 151)
Salad

Swap: Swap the Cheddar for Red Leicester.

Tenderise each chicken breast either using a tenderiser or grab a layer of clingfilm, cover the chicken and bash well with a rolling pin to flatten each breast. Season with salt and pepper, then dip into the beaten egg, then the panko breadcrumbs.

Place the coated chicken in a frying pan, spray with plenty of low-calorie cooking spray and fry for 8–10 minutes, flipping halfway and spraying again. Let it rest while you make your béchamel.

In a pan, heat the butter until melted, then mix in the flour. Once it's turned into a paste, keep on a low–medium heat, slowly adding a bit of milk at a time, whisking to remove any lumps. Keep gradually adding the milk until it forms a thick béchamel sauce (this takes about 5 minutes), then mix in the nutmeg and season with salt and pepper.

Place the breadcrumbed chicken on a lined baking tray, spread the béchamel over each chicken breast, then top with the Cheddar. Place under a hot grill until the cheese has melted and enjoy!

Air fryer method: Spray the breadcrumbed chicken with low-calorie cooking spray and air-fry at 200°C for 15–18 minutes, turning halfway and spraying with more low-calorie cooking spray.

KCAL	CARBS	PROTEIN	FAT		
446	24g	53g	15g	❄️	

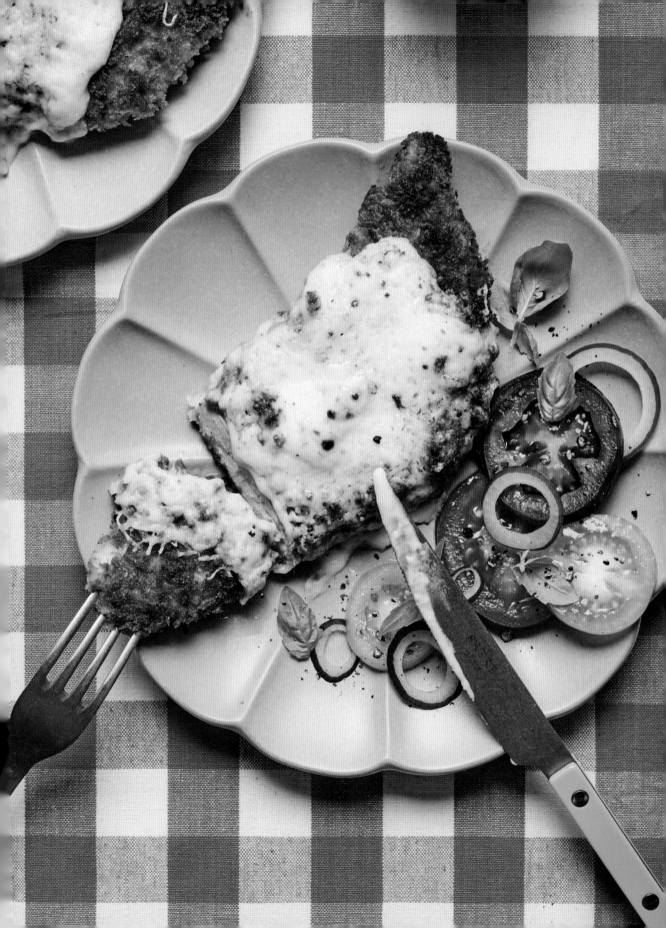

KUNG PAO KING PRAWNS

SERVES: 3 | **PREP:** 5 MINS | **COOK:** 10–12 MINS | DF

Juicy king prawns in a luscious, light batter, swimming in a sweet, sour and slightly spicy sauce and topped off with crunchy peanuts. A bold dish you'll love!

30g peanuts

Low-calorie cooking spray

2 different coloured peppers, diced

½ onion, diced

2.5cm piece of fresh ginger, peeled and minced

2 garlic cloves, minced

½ tsp chilli flakes

360g raw king prawns

2 tsp soy sauce

1 egg, beaten

40ml cornflour

Sliced spring onions, to serve (optional)

Sauce
4 tbsp oyster sauce

1 tbsp sriracha

2–3 tsp granulated or powdered sweetener

1 tsp rice vinegar

Side suggestion
Egg fried rice

Swaps: Don't fancy prawns? Swap for chicken or tofu and swap soy sauce for tamari to make this gluten-free.

Mix the sauce ingredients together and set aside.

In a large dry frying pan, fry the peanuts for a few minutes to toast, then remove and set aside.

Spray the same pan with low-calorie cooking spray and fry the peppers, onion, ginger, garlic and chilli flakes for a few minutes to soften, then remove and set aside.

Coat the prawns in soy sauce, dip into the beaten egg, then the cornflour. Fry for 2 minutes on each side or until cooked, spraying the prawns with plenty of low-calorie cooking spray.

Add the veg and peanuts back to the pan along with the sauce and cook on high until the sauce coats everything wonderfully.

Optional: Sprinkle with sliced spring onions to serve.

Air fryer method: Spray the battered prawns with low-calorie cooking spray and air-fry for 5–6 minutes or until cooked.

KCAL	CARBS	PROTEIN	FAT		
320	31g	31g	8g		

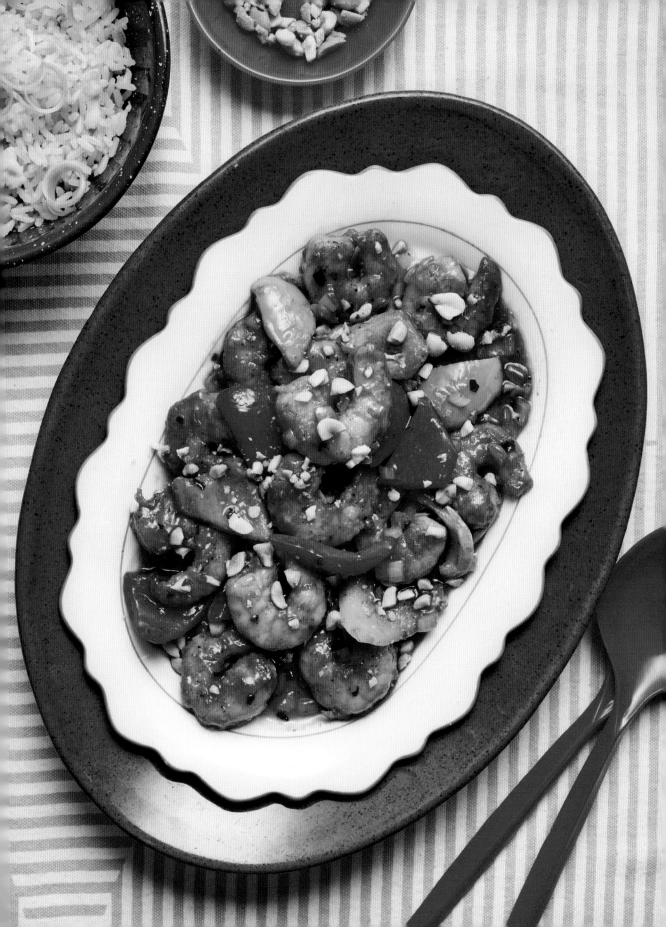

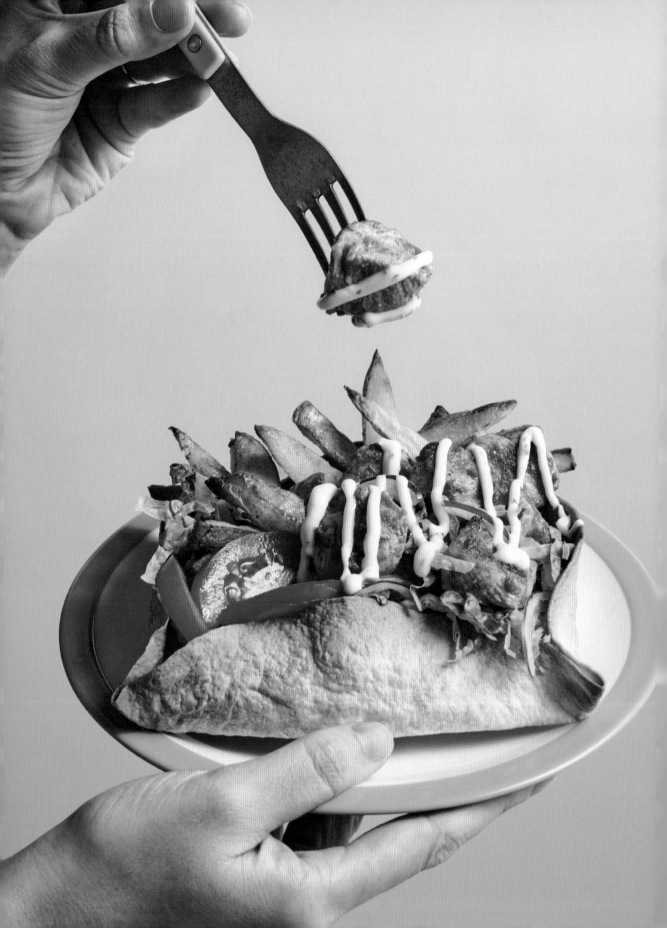

KEBAB FAKEAWAY BOX

SERVES: 2 | **PREP**: 5 MINS (+30 MINS MARINATING) | **COOK**: 6–8 MINS | NF

This fakeaway box will stop you from ringing up a takeaway as it has it all. Chicken tikka masala, homemade chips and a yummy salad. All finished off with drizzle of garlic mayonnaise.

2 chicken breasts, diced

Low-calorie cooking spray

2 tortilla wraps

200g homemade chips (page 151), cooked

2 handfuls of lettuce, sliced

1 tomato, sliced

2 slices of red onion

2 tbsp garlic mayonnaise

Marinade

1 tbsp tikka masala paste

1 heaped tbsp yogurt

2.5cm piece of fresh ginger, peeled and minced

1 garlic clove, minced

A pinch of salt and pepper

Swap: Use 1 tbsp garam masala if you can't find the tikka masala paste!

TIP: *If I'm feeling lazy, I use shop-bought chips!*

Preheat the oven to 180°C.

Mix all the marinade ingredients together in a bowl and add the diced chicken. Leave to marinate for at least 30 minutes. Spray a frying pan with low-calorie cooking spray and cook the chicken on a medium heat for 6–7 minutes or until cooked.

At the same time, press the tortillas in two rectangle dishes (or do one at a time) and cook in the oven for 6–8 minutes so that the tortillas hold their shape.

Place the chips to one side of each tortilla, then add the salad and chicken. Drizzle with 1 tablespoon of garlic mayo per kebab box and enjoy!

Air fryer method: Place the marinated chicken in foil and air-fry at 200°C for 10–15 minutes. Remove, then place the tortilla wrap in a dish or bowl that fits in your air fryer and air-fry for a couple of minutes.

KCAL	CARBS	PROTEIN	FAT		
459	51g	50g	6g		

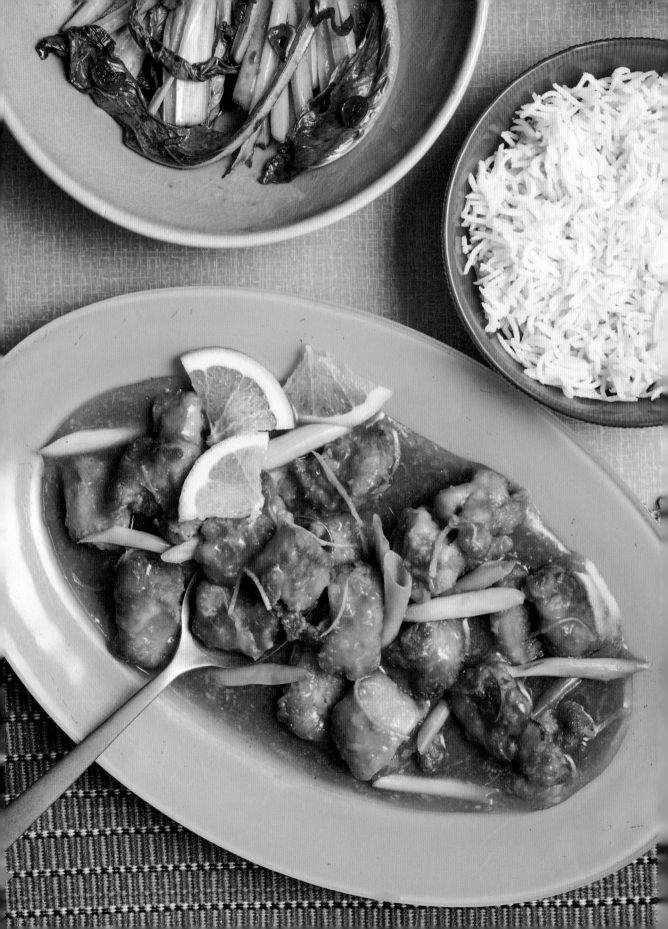

ORANGE CHICKEN

SERVES: 4 | **PREP**: 5 MINS | **COOK**: 22–24 MINS | DF + NF

This Chinese orange chicken dish is irresistible if you love a zesty, fragrant sauce and battered chicken. You even get an extra zesty kick from the organge peel, which takes the flavour to a whole new level.

6 large skinless chicken, boneless thighs, diced

2 tbsp light soy sauce

½ tsp white rice vinegar

2 egg whites, beaten

60g cornflour, plus 5g cornflour mixed with 1 tbsp water to make a slurry

Low-calorie cooking spray

2 garlic cloves, minced

2.5cm piece of fresh ginger, peeled and minced

Juice of 1½ medium oranges, plus peel of ½ orange

Sliced spring onions, to serve (optional)

Sauce

250ml chicken stock

1 tbsp light soy sauce

2 tbsp honey

Side suggestions

Boiled rice

Steamed veg

Swap: Use tamari instead of soy sauce to make this gluten-free.

Preheat the oven to 180°C.

Coat the chicken in the light soy sauce and white rice vinegar, then dip into the egg white and coat in 60g of the cornflour. Transfer to a lined baking tray, spray with low-calorie cooking spray and cook in the oven for 15–20 minutes, turning halfway.

Spray a large frying pan with low-calorie cooking spray and fry the garlic and ginger for 30–40 seconds, then add the sauce ingredients. Cook on a high heat for 1–2 minutes or until it starts to bubble, then pour in the orange juice and cornflour slurry. Mix well, then as soon as it thickens, stir in the orange peel and cooked chicken until it's all coated.

Optional: Finish with sliced spring onions.

Air fryer method: Spray the marinated chicken with low-calorie cooking spray and air-fry at 200°C for 10–15 minutes or until cooked, turning halfway.

KCAL	CARBS	PROTEIN	FAT		
342	26g	28g	14g	❄	

LEMON CHICKEN

SERVES: 4 | **PREP**: 5 MINS | **COOK**: 22–24 MINS | DF + NF

You just can't have lemon chicken without a beautiful batter! The thick, zesty sauce effortlessly coats the battered chicken pieces, and you get enough sauce to drizzle over at the end. Who doesn't love extra sauce?

6 large skinless, boneless chicken thighs, diced

2 tbsp light soy sauce

½ tsp white rice vinegar

2 egg whites, beaten

60g cornflour, plus 5g cornflour mixed with 1 tbsp water to make a slurry

Low-calorie cooking spray

2 garlic cloves, minced

2.5cm piece of fresh ginger, peeled and minced

Juice of 1½ lemons, plus zest of ½ lemon

Sliced spring onions, to serve (optional)

Sauce
250ml chicken stock

1 tbsp light soy sauce

2 tbsp honey

Side suggestions
Boiled rice

Steamed veg

Swap: Use tamari instead of soy sauce to make this gluten-free.

Preheat the oven to 180°C.

Marinade the chicken in the light soy sauce and white rice vinegar, then dip into the beaten egg white, then coat in 30g cornflour. Transfer to a lined baking tray, spray with low-calorie cooking spray and cook in the oven for 15–20 minutes, turning halfway.

Spray a large frying pan with low-calorie cooking spray and fry the garlic and ginger for 30–40 seconds, then add the sauce ingredients. Cook on a high heat for 1–2 minutes or until it starts to bubble, then pour in the lemon juice, zest and cornflour slurry. Mix well, then as soon as it thickens, stir in the cooked chicken until it's all coated and serve.

Optional: Finish with sliced spring onions.

Air fryer method: Spray the chicken with low-calorie cooking spray and air-fry at 200°C for 10–15 minutes or until cooked, turning halfway.

KCAL	CARBS	PROTEIN	FAT
336	15g	28g	14g

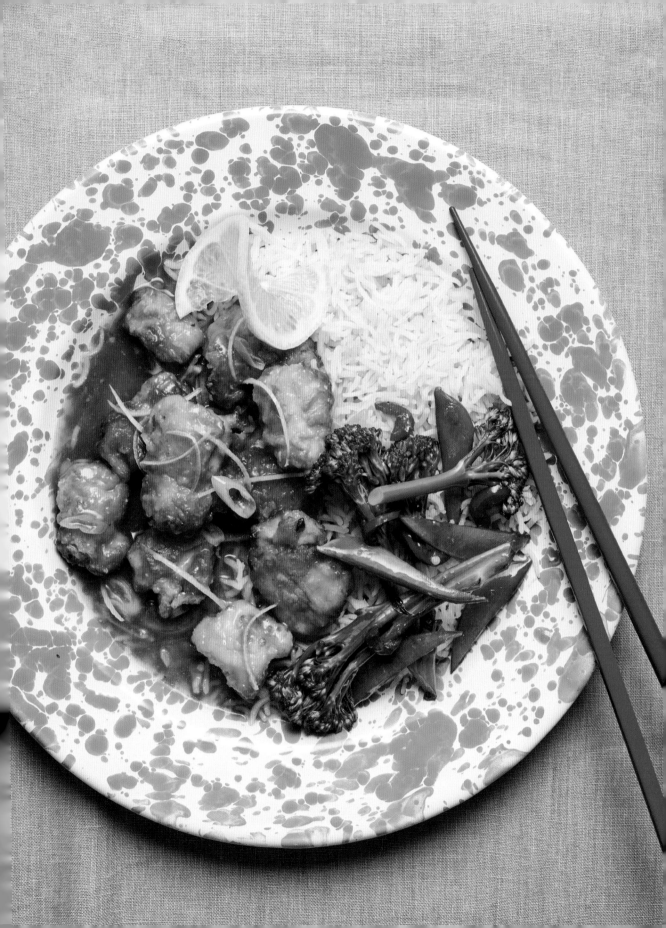

CHEESEBURGER CALZONE

SERVES: 2 | **PREP**: 2 MINS | **COOK**: 22–24 MINS | NF

Use the miracle two-ingredient dough to make this calzone extra special. Flour and yogurt make an incredible low-calorie dough, filled with all the flavours of a cheeseburger. But if you don't fancy that filling, you can simply use whatever ingredients you prefer.

Low-calorie
  cooking spray
½ medium onion,
  finely diced
250g lean beef mince
½ tsp English mustard
1 tbsp tomato purée
1 beef stock cube
50ml boiling water
45g shredded
  mozzarella
1 gherkin, sliced
1 tbsp burger sauce
½ medium onion,
  finely diced

Calzone base
100g self-raising
  flour, plus extra
  for dusting
150g 0% fat
  Greek yogurt
Pinch of salt

Side suggestion
Side salad

TIP: *This recipe only works with thick, Greek yogurt – none of the natural yogurt stuff!*

Preheat the oven to 180°C.

Spray a pan with low-calorie cooking spray and fry the onion for a few minutes to soften. Add the beef mince and fry for a further 3–4 minutes. Mix in the English mustard, tomato purée, crumble over the beef stock cube and add the boiling water. Cook on a medium–high heat for 1–2 minutes, then let it cool.

Next, in a large bowl, mix the flour, yogurt and salt together until it forms a dough. Cut in half and then roll out each piece on a floured surface to roughly the thickness of a pound coin.

Place the doughs on a lined baking tray. Place the filling on one side of each dough, then add the cheese and gherkin slices and drizzle over the burger sauce. Fold the dough over to form a calzone, twisting the edges to enclose (I use YouTube for the technique!).

Bake in the oven for 16–18 minutes and enjoy!

Air fryer method: Air-fry the calzone at 190°C for 10–12 minutes.

KCAL	CARBS	PROTEIN	FAT
486	45g	44g	14g

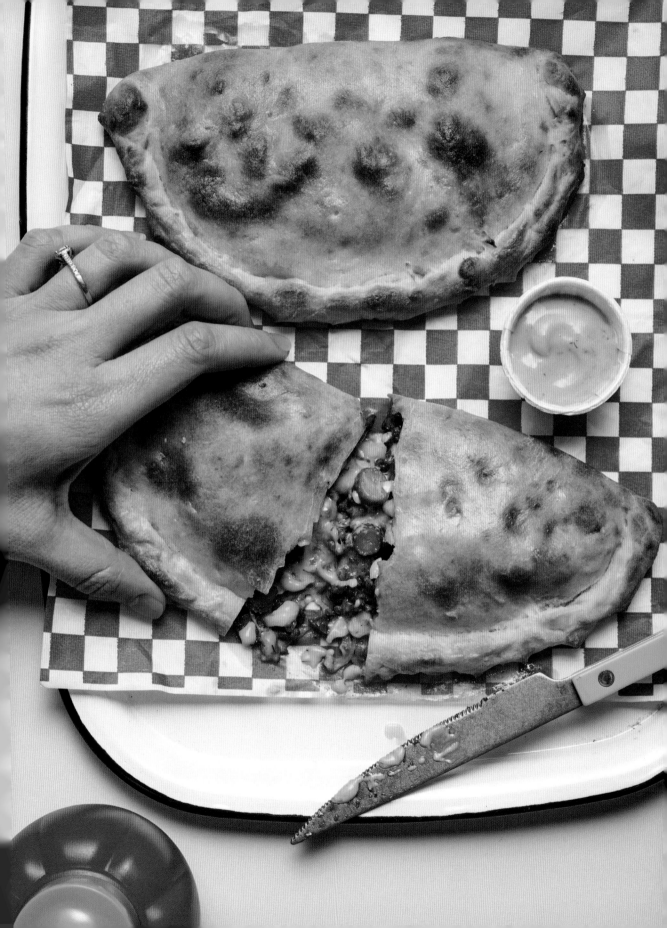

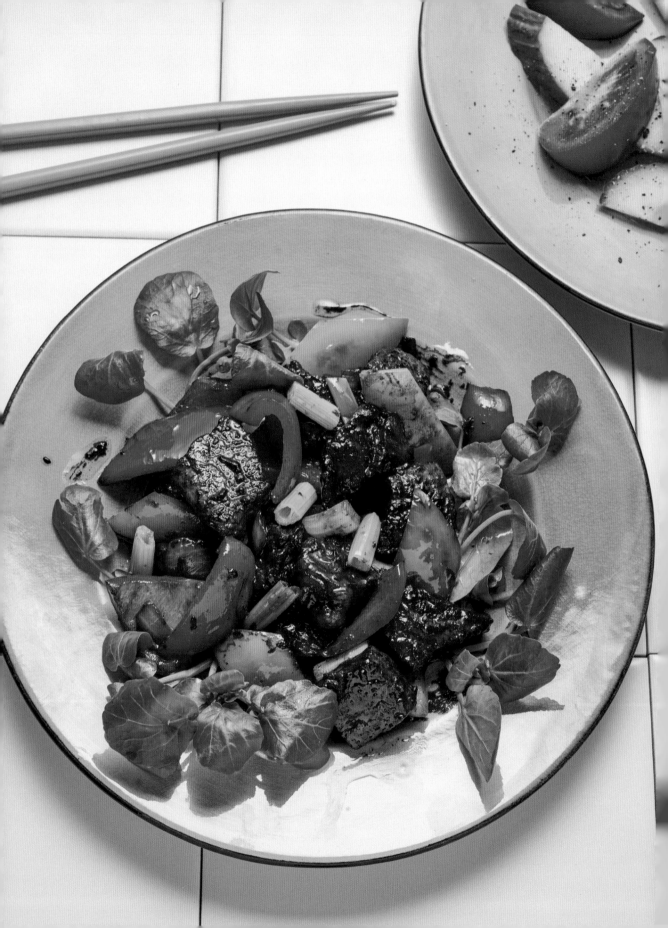

SHAKING BEEF

SERVES: 4 | **PREP**: 5 MINS (+30 MINS MARINATING) | **COOK**: 8–10 MINS | GF

Shaking and tossing the beef in a hot wok or pan is what gives this dish its name. Super flavourful sautéed beef mixed with a heap of veg, sits on a fresh bed of watercress, cucumber and tomatoes, which pairs flawlessly with the beef.

4 x 200g rump or sirloin steaks, fat removed and cubed

Low-calorie cooking spray

1 large onion, diced

1 red pepper, diced

1 orange pepper, diced

2 spring onions, diced

2 tsp low-fat butter (optional)

4 handfuls of watercress

4 tomatoes, sliced

10cm piece of cucumber, sliced

Marinade

3 tbsp oyster sauce

2 tbsp soy sauce

1 tbsp dark soy sauce

2–3 tbsp granulated or powdered sweetener

3 garlic cloves, minced

Good pinch of black pepper

Swaps: Don't fancy serving it with salad? Swap it for rice and use tamari instead of soy sauce to make this gluten-free.

Mix all the marinade ingredients together and marinate the beef for at least 30 minutes or overnight for a more intense flavour.

Spray a pan with low-calorie cooking spray and fry the onion, peppers and spring onions for 5–6 minutes until softened. (I like to add a splash of water near the end to soften them further.) Remove from the pan and set aside.

In the same pan, fry the beef in more low-calorie cooking spray for 3–4 minutes on a medium–high heat, pouring over any remaining marinade for the last minute of cooking, along with the butter (if using).

Mix in the cooked veg, then add the mixture to the top of a bed of watercress, with the tomatoes and cucumber on the side.

Optional: Add 2 teaspoons of butter to the beef for the last minute of frying for a true Vietnamese experience.

KCAL	CARBS	PROTEIN	FAT	
374	17g	54g	10g	❄

CROWD-PLEASERS

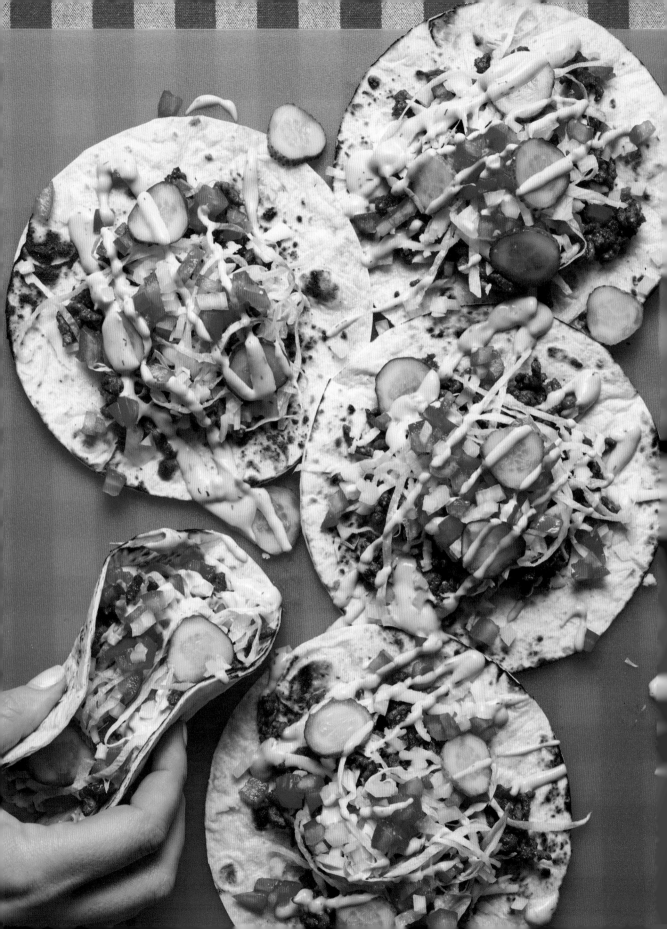

BURGER TACOS

SERVES: 2 | **PREP**: 5 MINS | **COOK**: 8–10 MINS | DF + NF

If you're in the mood for Mexican but also in the mood for burgers, why not have both?! When I made these the first time, I ate a second portion without even batting an eyelid.

Low-calorie
  cooking spray
⅓ medium onion,
  finely diced
240g lean beef mince
1 beef stock cube
20g tomato purée
½ tsp English mustard
½ tsp garlic granules
6 mini tortilla wraps
2 large handfuls
  of iceberg
  lettuce, sliced
2 tomatoes,
  finely diced
40g shredded
  mozzarella (optional)
2–3 tbsp burger sauce
2–3 gherkins, sliced

Spray a frying pan with low-calorie cooking spray and fry half of the finely diced onion for 2–3 minutes to soften, then add the mince.

Fry for a further 4–5 minutes, then crumble over the stock cube and add a couple of tablespoons of water, the tomato purée, mustard and garlic granules. Mix well and cook on a high heat for 30 seconds.

Lightly toast the mini tortilla wraps, then divide the lettuce, tomatoes, mince and remaining onion between them. Add the gherkins then drizzle over the burger sauce and enjoy.

Optional: Melt some mozzarella on the mince before adding the onion and burger sauce.

KCAL	CARBS	PROTEIN	FAT	
495	57g	36g	13g	❄️

MOUSSAKA

SERVES: 4 | **PREP:** 5 MINS | **COOK:** 25–30 MINS | NF

A Greek classic and instant crowd-pleaser. I've made it super simple
with the layers you all know and love, but kept the calories down.

2 medium aubergines

1–2 tsp salt

Low-calorie
   cooking spray

1 red onion,
   finely diced

3 garlic cloves, minced

500g lean beef mince

400g tin chopped
   tomatoes

250g passata

20g tomato purée

A pinch of ground
   cinnamon

2 bay leaves

Salt and pepper

Béchamel

15g low-fat butter

15g plain flour

150ml semi-
   skimmed milk

A good pinch of
   black pepper

A pinch of nutmeg

40g Parmesan, grated

2 egg yolks

Side suggestions

Greek salad or
   mixed leaves

TIP: *Add more
cinnamon and
nutmeg for a
greater Greek
flavour!*

Preheat the oven to 200°C.

Slice the aubergines lengthways into 3mm slices, place in a
large bowl, coat with a good few pinches of salt and set aside.

Spray a large pan with low-calorie cooking spray and fry the
onion and garlic for a few minutes to soften, then add the beef
mince and fry for a further few minutes. Add the remaining
ingredients and cook on a medium heat for 5–6 minutes.

Meanwhile, make the béchamel. In a small pan, melt the butter,
then mix in the flour. On a low–medium heat, gradually pour
in the milk until the sauce has thickened. Mix in the pepper,
nutmeg and half of the grated Parmesan. Take it off the heat,
then mix in the egg yolks until well combined.

Squeeze out any moisture from the aubergine or use kitchen
paper to pat dry. Spray a frying pan or griddle pan, if you
have one, with plenty of low-calorie cooking spray and fry
the aubergine slices on a high heat for 1–2 minutes each
side or until charred.

Place the aubergine at the bottom of an ovenproof dish, then
layer over the beef mixture (remembering to take out the bay
leaves!), then the béchamel. Scatter over the remaining Parmesan
and cook in the oven for 16–18 minutes or until the top is a lovely
dark brown colour. Let it rest for 5 minutes, then serve.

KCAL	CARBS	PROTEIN	FAT	
348	18g	37g	15g	

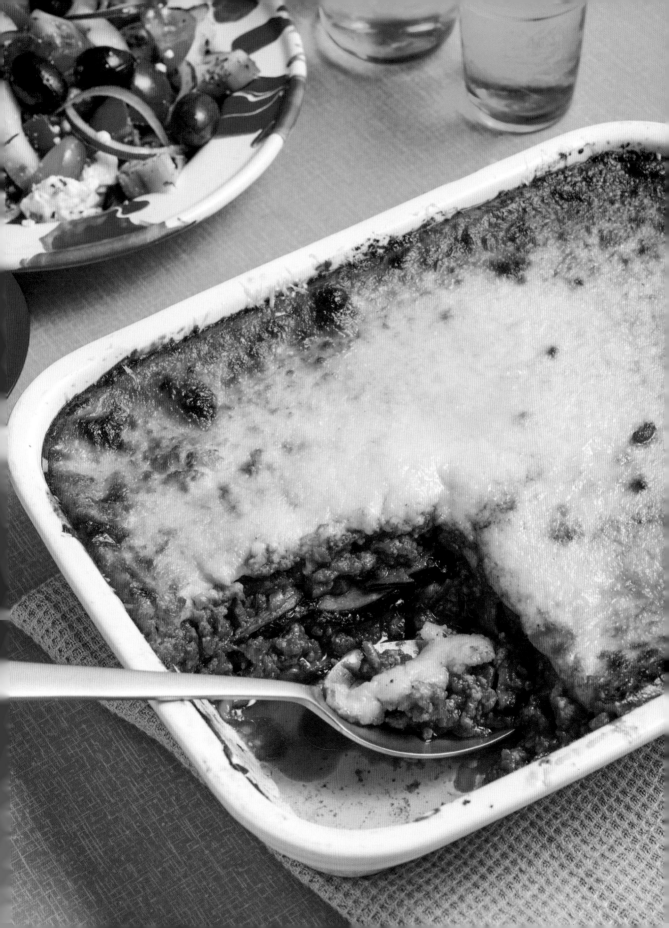

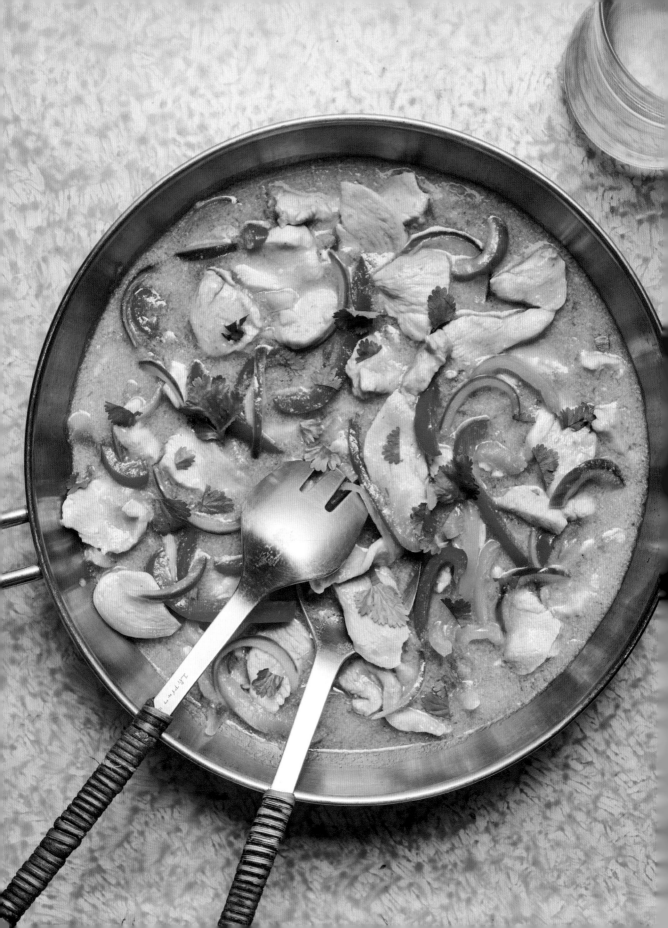

LEMONGRASS COCONUT CHICKEN

SERVES: 2 | **PREP**: 5 MINS | **COOK**: 10–12 MINS | GF + DF + NF

A vibrant and citrussy lemon-flavoured chicken dish infused in a creamy coconut sauce.

Low-calorie
  cooking spray
2 garlic cloves, minced
1 heaped tsp
  lemongrass paste
½ red onion, sliced
½ red pepper, sliced
½ yellow pepper,
  sliced
2 chicken breasts,
  sliced
200ml reduced-fat
  coconut milk
200ml chicken stock
A few dashes of
  fish sauce
1 tsp granulated
  or powdered
  sweetener
2 tsp cornflour mixed
  with 1–2 tbsp water
  to make a slurry
Coriander leaves, to
  finish (optional)

Side suggestion
Basmati rice

Spray a large pan with low-calorie cooking spray and fry the garlic, lemongrass paste and all the veg for 2–3 minutes to soften, then add all the remaining ingredients, except the cornflour slurry.

Simmer on a low heat for 5–6 minutes, then mix in the cornflour slurry. Cook on a high heat for a few more minutes to allow the sauce to thicken and ensure the chicken is cooked. Serve and enjoy!

Optional: Finish with a sprinkle of coriander for a fresh flavour pop.

KCAL	CARBS	PROTEIN	FAT	
316	14g	42g	10g	❄

GARLIC BREAD PERI-PERI CHICKEN BURGER

SERVES: 2 | **PREP:** 2 MINS (+30 MINS MARINATING) | **COOK:** 10 MINS | GF + NF

This burger was inspired by a flame-grilled peri-peri chicken joint that you all know and love. Tender pieces of peri-peri chicken with Perinaise sauce, grilled slices of halloumi and salad in between slices of heavenly garlic bread. You will LOVE it.

2 chicken breasts

3 tbsp peri-peri marinade

Low-calorie cooking spray

60g light halloumi, sliced

4 tsp Perinaise sauce

A handful of lettuce

1 tomato, sliced

Salt and pepper

Garlic bread

4 tsp low-fat butter

½ tsp parsley, finely diced

2 garlic cloves, minced

2 gluten-free ciabatta rolls, sliced

Side suggestions

Homemade chips (see page 151) or spicy rice with corn on the cob

TIP: *If you don't have Perinaise sauce to hand, mix peri-peri marinade with light mayo for the same thing!*

Butterfly both chicken breasts, then season with salt, pepper and 2 tablespoons of peri-peri marinade. If you can, leave it to marinate for 30 minutes, but the longer the better.

Spray a frying pan with low-calorie cooking spray and fry the chicken on a medium heat for 3 minutes each side, then crank up the heat to high and pour over the remaining 1 tablespoon of marinade. Fry for a further 30 seconds–1 minute, then leave the chicken to rest for 3 minutes.

In the same pan, while the chicken is resting, fry the halloumi for a few minutes, flipping halfway until browned. Then, mix the butter, parsley and garlic together, and spread over each top slice of ciabatta roll. Place in a hot frying pan for 30 seconds–1 minute to lightly brown.

Spread the Perinaise sauce over the bottom slices of the ciabatta rolls, then layer with the lettuce, tomato, halloumi and chicken. Top with the garlic bread top and enjoy!

KCAL	CARBS	PROTEIN	FAT
476	27g	51g	17g

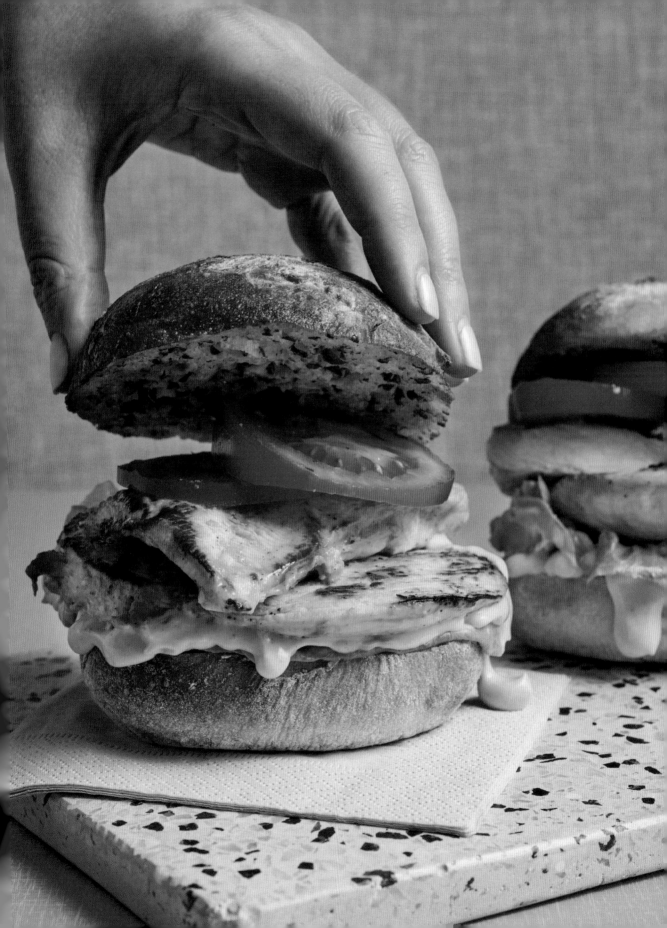

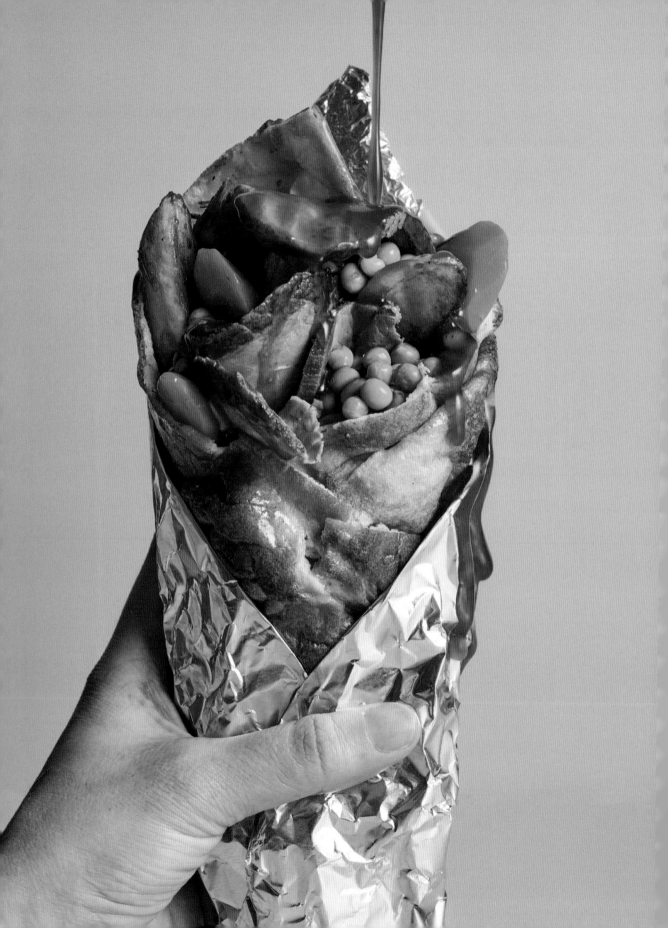

ROAST BEEF YORKSHIRE PUDDING WRAP

SERVES: 2 | **PREP:** 5 MINS (+30 MINS RESTING) | **COOK:** 20–22 MINS | NF

My death-row meal has got to be anything with Yorkshire pudding, so if you're like me, you need to try this recipe immediately. It's perfect if you have leftover roast beef or chicken, but you can cheat and use shop-bought. Delicious with homemade crispy roasties and veg crammed in, oh and don't forget a boatload of gravy.

40g plain flour

2 eggs

135ml semi-skimmed milk

1 medium potato, peeled

Low-calorie cooking spray

½ tsp dried rosemary

200g cooked beef, sliced

1 carrot, sliced and boiled

70g peas, cooked

100ml gravy

Salt and pepper

Swap: You can swap the beef for chicken, sausages or even a nut roast.

Preheat the oven to 200°C.

Whisk the flour, eggs and milk together well, making sure there's no lumps, then place in the fridge for at least 30 minutes.

Slice the potato into wedges, then boil the wedges in boiling salted water for 5–6 minutes until they start to soften. Drain and shake so they fluff up, then place on a lined baking tray. Spray with low-calorie cooking spray, then season with a good pinch of salt, pepper and the rosemary.

Heat 2 square-shaped ovenproof dishes with plenty of low-calorie cooking spray in the oven for 8 minutes, then pour in the batter you made earlier (give it a good stir first!), along with the wedges on a separate oven shelf.

Cook in the oven for 14 minutes, remove the Yorkshire puddings and make sure the potato wedges are cooked through. If not flip and place back in the oven until cooked and crispy.

Remove the Yorkshire puddings from the dishes and use a spatula to press them flat. Divide the beef, carrot, peas and potatoes between the two Yorkshire pudding wraps, then pour over the gravy or keep it for pouring over once the wraps are assembled.

Carefully roll up the wraps and secure them with foil or parchment paper, then dig in!

KCAL	CARBS	PROTEIN	FAT	
473	48g	45g	11g	❄️

RAID THE FRIDGE CRUSTLESS QUICHE

SERVES: 4 | **PREP**: 5 MINS | **COOK**: 25–30 MINS | GF + NF

The name says it all. Use whatever ingredients you have to hand – whether that's veggies or meat – to make this quiche to your liking.

6 eggs

115ml semi-skimmed milk

60g reduced-fat Cheddar, grated

100g ham slices, diced

4 bacon medallions, cooked

5 mushrooms, sliced

1 tomato, sliced

85g tinned sweetcorn, drained

Low-calorie cooking spray

Salt and pepper

Swaps: As the recipe name suggests, use whatever you've got in your fridge for the filling, including any cooked meat.

TIP: You can use a 12-hole Yorkshire pudding tray for bite-sized quiches but cook for only 15–20 minutes.

Preheat the oven to 180°C.

Whisk the eggs and milk together in a large bowl, then stir in half the Cheddar, the meat and veg, then a good pinch of salt and pepper.

Spray a 20–24cm quiche or pie dish with plenty of low-calorie cooking spray and pour in the quiche mixture. Top with the remaining cheese and bake in the oven for 25–30 minutes.

KCAL	CARBS	PROTEIN	FAT	
226	6g	27g	10g	❄

HONEY-CHIPOTLE BEEF CHOW MEIN

SERVES: 2 | **PREP:** 2 MINS | **COOK:** 8–10 MINS | GF + DF + NF

This is sweet, smoky goodness right here. The honey really cools down the heat of the chipotle and beef stock makes this noodle dish extra rich and beefy.

Low-calorie
  cooking spray
1 medium onion, sliced
1 coloured pepper,
  sliced
250g lean beef mince
A handful of
  beansprouts
100g dried egg
  noodles, cooked

Sauce
1 tsp chipotle paste
1 heaped tbsp honey
2 tbsp tomato purée
1 beef stock cube
60ml water

To serve (optional)
A squeeze of lime juice
Finely chopped
  fresh coriander

Mix all the sauce ingredients together in a jug or bowl.

Spray a large frying pan with low-calorie cooking spray and fry the onion and pepper for a few minutes to soften, then add the beef mince. Fry for a further 3–4 minutes or until the beef is cooked, adding the beansprouts for the last minute of cooking.

Pour in half of the sauce, mix well, then add the cooked egg noodles and remaining sauce. Make sure everything is coated well and serve.

Optional: Add a squeeze of lime juice and finely chopped coriander to serve.

KCAL	CARBS	PROTEIN	FAT	
445	56g	37g	8g	❄

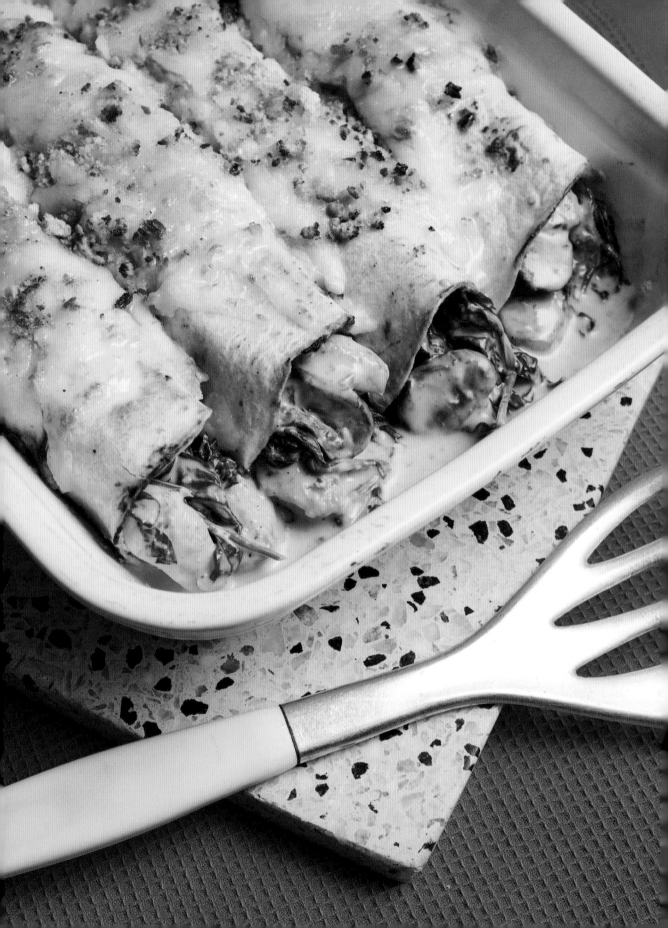

CHICKEN ALFREDO ENCHILADAS WITH A CRUNCHY CRUMB

SERVES: 4 | **PREP:** 5 MINS | **COOK:** 20–25 MINS | NF

Creamy Alfredo-inspired chicken enchiladas that will send you into euphoria. To top them off, and for a real texture sensation, I've added a crunchy breadcrumb coating.

4 chicken breasts, diced

1 tsp onion granules

½ tsp garlic granules

1 tsp Italian mixed herbs

Low-calorie cooking spray

10–12 mushrooms, sliced

3 handfuls of spinach

4 tortilla wraps

100g reduced-fat mozzarella, grated

10g panko breadcrumbs

Salt and pepper

Alfredo sauce

180ml semi-skimmed milk

100g reduced-fat soft cheese

15g Parmesan, grated

1 tsp Italian mixed herbs

Preheat the oven to 180°C.

Season the diced chicken with the onion granules, garlic granules, Italian herbs and a pinch of salt and pepper. Spray a large pan with low-calorie cooking spray and cook the chicken for 4–5 minutes, then add the mushrooms and fry for a further few minutes.

Add the alfredo sauce ingredients to the pan and mix well. Cook on a high heat for 1–2 minutes, then stir in the spinach. Divide the chicken mixture equally between the wraps, leaving the leftover sauce in the pan, and roll up the wraps.

Spread a small amount of the leftover sauce over the bottom of an ovenproof dish, then place the rolled wraps on top lengthways. Pour over any remaining sauce, then scatter over the mozzarella and the breadcrumbs.

Cook in the oven for 12–14 minutes.

TIP: *This dish goes super dry when reheating due to the Parmesan, so eat it all on the day!*

KCAL	CARBS	PROTEIN	FAT	❄
425	31g	56g	8g	

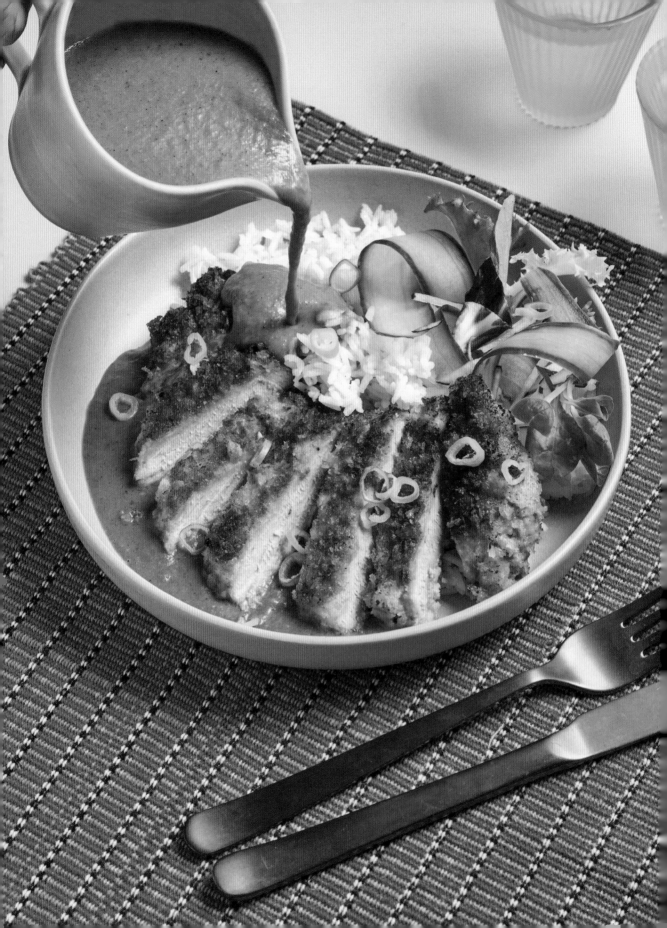

PORK KATSU CURRY

SERVES: 4 | **PREP**: 5 MINS | **COOK**: 10–12 MINS | DF + NF

The rich katsu sauce, the crispy fried breaded pork . . . it's comforting, filling and flavoursome. I always have spare sauce in the freezer ready to go for when I fancy making this.

4 lean pork steaks (480g)

1 egg, beaten

40g panko breadcrumbs

Low-calorie cooking spray

Salt and pepper

Katsu sauce

3 medium carrots, sliced

1 medium onion, sliced

2.5cm piece of fresh ginger, minced

2 garlic cloves, peeled and minced

1 tbsp curry powder of your choice

1 tsp garam masala

1 tbsp honey

2 tsp soy sauce

550ml chicken stock

Side suggestions

Boiled rice

Side salad

Swap: If you don't fancy pork, swap it for chicken or make it veggie by using sliced sweet potato and veggie stock!

Use a tenderiser or cover the pork steaks with clingfilm and bash with a rolling pin to tenderise.

Season the pork steaks with salt and pepper, dip into the beaten egg, then into the panko breadcrumbs. Spray a pan with low-calorie cooking spray and cook the coated pork for 3–4 minutes on each side. Remove from the pan and leave to rest for at least 3 minutes.

While the pork steaks are frying, spray a separate pan with low-calorie cooking spray and fry the carrots and onion for 3–4 minutes until softened. Add the ginger, garlic, curry powder and garam masala and fry for a further minute.

Add the remaining katsu sauce ingredients, mix well and simmer for 6–8 minutes, then blend in a food processor or with a hand blender until smooth. Serve the pork coated in the katsu sauce.

Air fryer method: Spray the coated pork with low-calorie cooking spray and air-fry at 190°C for 7 minutes before flipping and spraying with more low-calorie cooking spray and air-frying for a further 7 minutes.

KCAL	CARBS	PROTEIN	FAT		
476	20g	35g	29g	❄	

IRRESISTIBLE LAMB CHOPS WITH BUTTERY SWEET POTATO MASH

SERVES: 2 | PREP: 5 MINS | COOK: 24–26 MINS | GF + NF

If I could eat a plate of lamb chops, I would. These are heavily seasoned to make every mouthful a flavour explosion. Team with a buttery sweet potato mash, which pairs with the lamb chops like bread with butter.

4 lean lamb chops

2 medium sweet potatoes, peeled and diced

1 tbsp low-fat butter, plus a knob (optional)

Low-calorie cooking spray

1–2 tbsp finely chopped fresh parsley

Salt and pepper

Marinade

1 tbsp honey

½ tsp onion granules

½ tsp garlic granules

1 tsp paprika

½ tsp chilli powder of your choice

1 tsp English or Dijon mustard

Side suggestion

Grilled Tenderstem broccoli

Mix all the marinade ingredients together in a bowl and add the lamb chops. Leave to marinate while you make your sweet potato mash.

Boil the diced sweet potatoes in salted water for 20 minutes or until tender, then mash. Mix in the butter and season with a pinch of salt and pepper.

Spray a deep pan with low-calorie cooking spray and fry the lamb chops on a high heat for 1–2 minutes on each side (I like mine pink in the middle) or until cooked to your liking. Top with fresh parsley and serve with your sweet potato mash.

Optional: Add a knob of butter to the pan once the lamb chops have finished cooking and baste for a flavour pop.

KCAL	CARBS	PROTEIN	FAT
474	35g	44g	19g

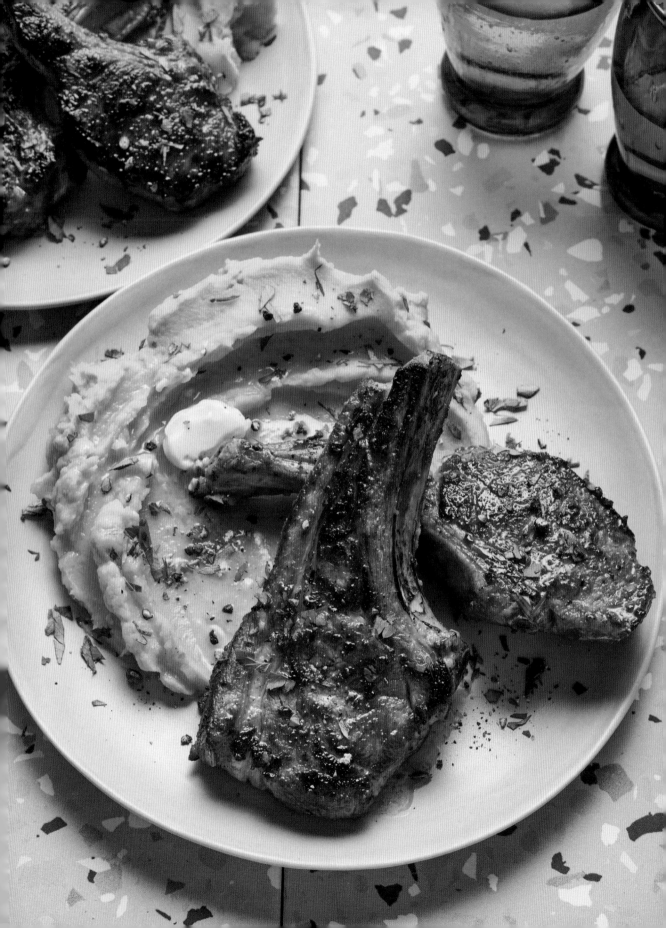

CREAMY CHICKEN, LEEK AND MUSHROOM FILO PIE

SERVES: 4 | **PREP:** 5 MINS | **COOK:** 21–23 MINS | NF

A pie isn't complete without pastry, but instead of using a calorie-filled pastry like shortcrust, I've opted for a lighter filo that goes so well with the creamy chicken, leek and mushroom filling.

1 tbsp low-fat butter

2 medium leeks, sliced

8 chestnut mushrooms, sliced

4 chicken breasts, diced

60ml reduced-fat crème fraîche

100ml chicken stock

A handful of spinach (optional)

2 tsp cornflour mixed with 2–3 tbsp water to make a slurry

3 sheets of filo pastry

Low-calorie cooking spray

Salt and pepper

Side suggestions
Mashed potato
Green vegetables

Preheat the oven to 180°C.

Fry the leeks and mushrooms in the butter in a large pan for 4–5 minutes to soften. Remove from the pan and set aside, then add the diced chicken and season with salt and pepper. Fry for 5–6 minutes until nearly cooked.

Return the veg to the pan, then mix in the crème fraîche, stock and spinach (if using) until well combined. Mix in the cornflour slurry to thicken the sauce, then add a pinch of black pepper and transfer to a pie dish.

One at a time, scrunch up the filo pastry sheets and place on top of the mixture. Spray with low-calorie cooking spray and bake in the oven for 10–12 minutes until the filo is golden brown.

Optional: Sometimes I like to add a handful of spinach to the pie when mixing in the stock.

KCAL	CARBS	PROTEIN	FAT	
319	21g	44g	6g	❄

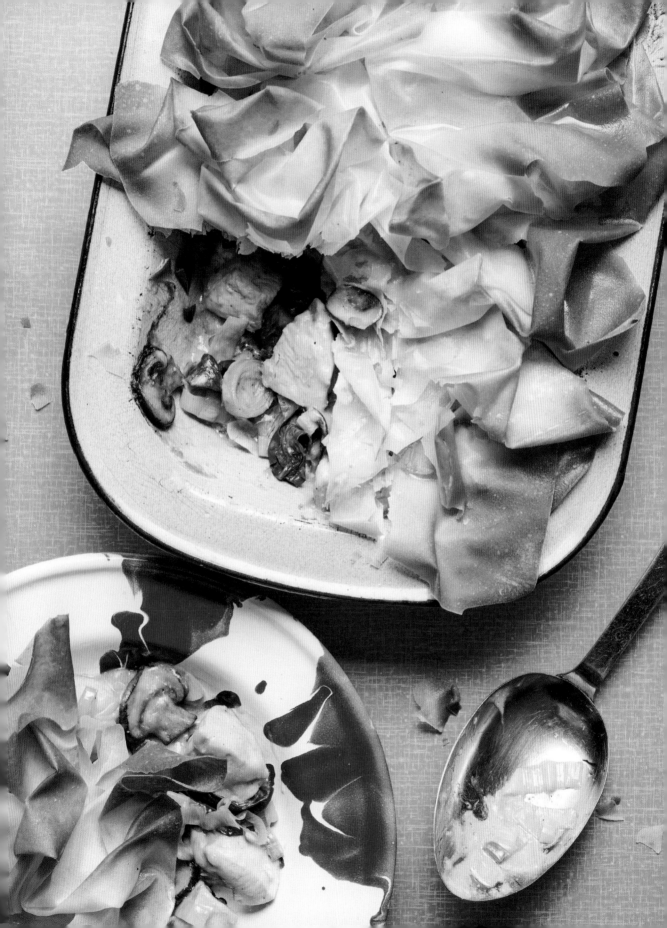

EASY PEASY CHICKEN KIEVS

SERVES: 2 | **PREP:** 5 MINS + 15 MINS FREEZE | **COOK:** 25–30 MINS | NF

A breadcrumbed chicken breast filled with seductive garlic butter.
When you take your first bite the garlic butter will flow out like
lava and is perfectly paired with creamy mash and veg.

30g low-fat butter

1 tbsp finely chopped
 fresh parsley

3 garlic cloves, minced

2 chicken breasts

1 egg, beaten

20g panko
 breadcrumbs

Low-calorie
 cooking spray

Salt and pepper

Side suggestions

Homemade chips
 (see page 151) or
 mashed potato

Any veg you like

Preheat the oven to 190°C.

Mix the butter, parsley and garlic together. Place in clingfilm, wrap up tight and freeze for at least 15 minutes, then slice in half.

Season the chicken breasts with salt and pepper, then using a sharp knife, make a deep pocket at the top of both chicken breasts. Placing a piece of garlic butter firmly in each pocket. Dip the chicken into the beaten egg, then panko breadcrumbs. Spray a lined baking tray with low-calorie cooking spray.

Place the chicken kievs on the tray with the pockets facing up, spray with low-calorie cooking spray and cook in the oven for 25–30 minutes or until cooked.

Air fryer method: Place the kievs in the air fryer with the pockets facing up, spray with low-calorie cooking spray and air-fry at 180°C for 20–25 minutes or until cooked.

KCAL	CARBS	PROTEIN	FAT		
313	8g	45g	11g		

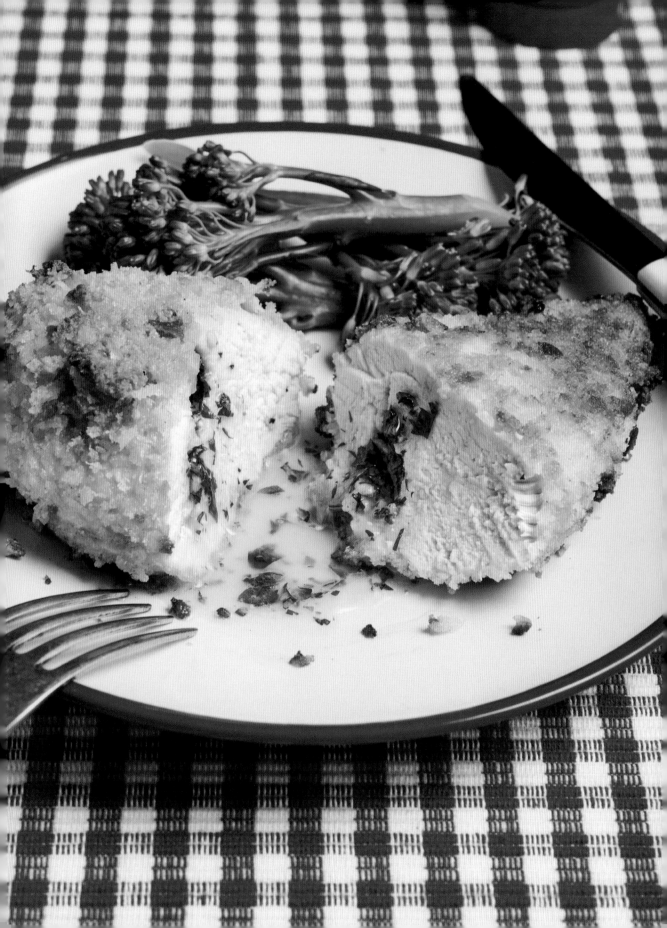

BUDGET
BANGERS

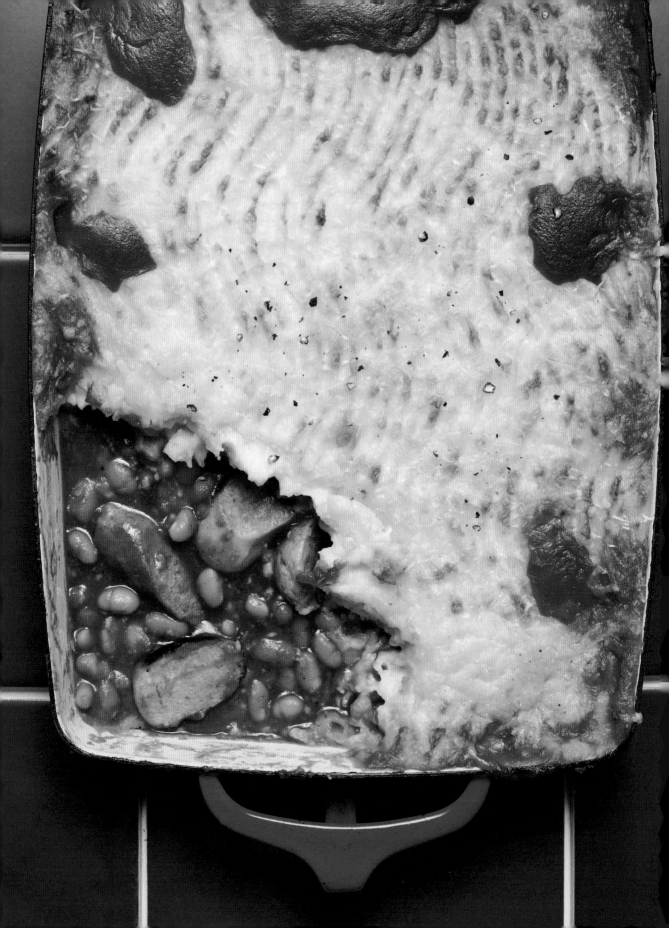

BBQ COWBOY PIE

SERVES: 4 | **PREP:** 5 MINS | **COOK:** 25–30 MINS | GF + NF

This is ridiculously cheap and easy to make, and if you have kids, they are going to LOVE it! It's simply sausages, BBQ beans and mash topped with cheese and baked in the oven. Actually, I take that back, you're going to love it, too!

2 medium potatoes, peeled and diced

165ml semi-skimmed milk

1 tbsp low-fat butter

A pinch of black pepper (optional)

Low-calorie cooking spray

8 reduced-fat pork sausages

2 x 400g tins reduced-sugar baked beans

4 tbsp BBQ sauce

80g reduced-fat Cheddar, grated

Side suggestions

Cooked peas or carrots

Swaps: If you're gluten intolerant swap in gluten-free sausages and BBQ sauce.

Preheat the oven to 180°C.

Boil the diced potatoes in salted water for 15 minutes or until tender. Drain, then add the milk and butter, plus black pepper (if using), and mash until it's creamy with no lumps.

Meanwhile, spray a large pan with low-calorie cooking spray and fry the sausages on a medium heat for 7–8 minutes. Slice the sausages into bite-sized pieces and add to the bottom of a large ovenproof dish.

Add the baked beans and BBQ sauce, mixing well with the sausages, then add a sprinkle of cheese over the top of the mixture, smooth over the mash, then add the remaining cheese.

Cook in the oven for 10–15 minutes or until the cheese is golden and serve.

Optional: Add a pinch of black pepper to the mash.

KCAL	CARBS	PROTEIN	FAT	
499	54g	32g	16g	

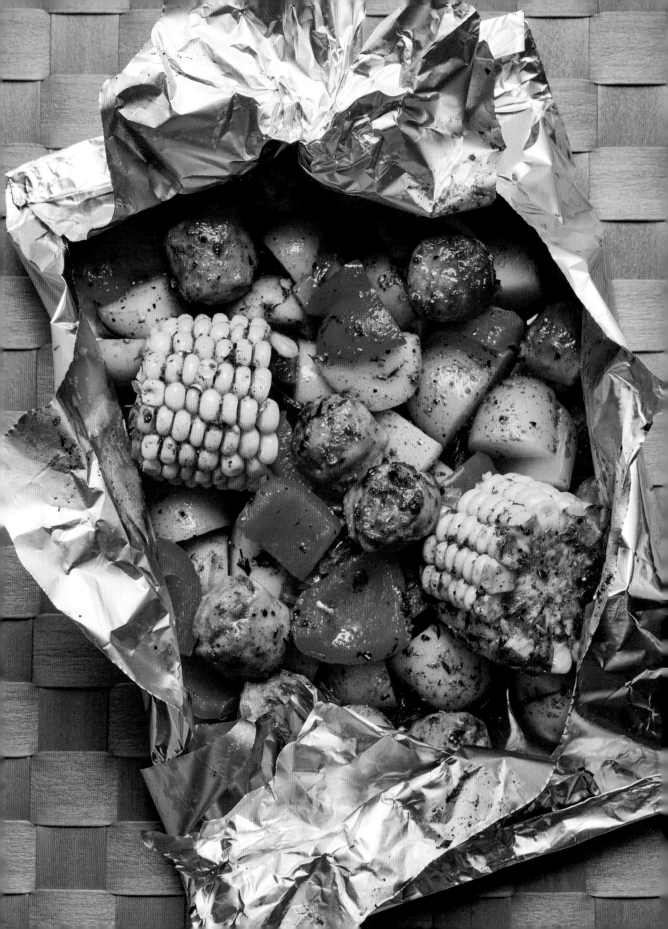

SMOKY SAUSAGE FOIL PARCELS

SERVES: 4 | **PREP**: 5 MINS | **COOK**: 20–25 MINS | GF + NF

Whack all the ingredients into foil, wrap up tightly, then cook and BOOM. You've got yourself the easiest dinner you'll ever make.

2½ tbsp low-fat butter, melted

4 tsp Cajun seasoning

½ red onion, diced

2 red peppers, diced

2 corn on the cobs, sliced into 5cm discs

400g new potatoes, quartered

200g reduced-fat smoked pork sausages, sliced

1–2 tbsp finely chopped fresh parsley

Salt and pepper

Swaps: Swap to pork or chicken sausages but fry them for a few minutes on a high heat before adding to the foil bags. If gluten intolerant swap the sausages for gluten-free ones.

Preheat the oven to 200°C.

Mix the melted butter with the Cajun seasoning and a good pinch of salt and pepper, then set aside.

Add the red onion, peppers, corn, potatoes and sausages to the middle of 4 large pieces of foil, then pour the seasoned melted butter evenly between each of the bags.

Wrap up each bag tightly so that the ingredients are fully enclosed, then cook in the oven for 20–25 minutes or until the potatoes are tender. Finish off with a sprinkle of fresh parsley.

Air fryer method: In the foil bags, air-fry at 200°C for 20–25 minutes or until the potatoes are tender.

KCAL	CARBS	PROTEIN	FAT		
320	31g	13g	16g		

BEEF PEPPER RICE

SERVES: 2 | **PREP**: 2 MINS | **COOK**: 5 MINS | NF

If you have ever been to Japan, there is a popular fast-food chain that popularised this beef pepper rice. It's super simple: just sliced beef, rice, corn, green onion and a sweet and salty sauce to drizzle over while it cooks. Mix in a knob of butter and it just melts in your mouth.

200g sirloin steak, fat removed then thinly sliced

200g tinned sweetcorn

100g basmati rice, cooked

1 tsp low-fat butter

1 tsp black pepper

2 spring onions, sliced

Sauce

2 tsp oyster sauce

2 tbsp soy sauce

1 tbsp honey

2 garlic cloves, minced

Swap: Use tamari instead of soy sauce to make this gluten-free.

TIP: *Any steak will work as long as it's sliced into flat thin slices.*

Mix all the sauce ingredients together and set aside.

In a large frying pan, add the sliced steak around the outside of the pan, then the sweetcorn and the cooked rice in the centre. Put the butter over the rice, along with the black pepper and spring onions.

Without stirring, fry for about 2 minutes on a medium heat, then pour over the sauce. Give everything a good stir and fry for a further 2–3 minutes or until the steak is cooked to your liking.

Optional: Add another piece of steak for extra protein.

KCAL	CARBS	PROTEIN	FAT	❄
393	47g	31g	9g	

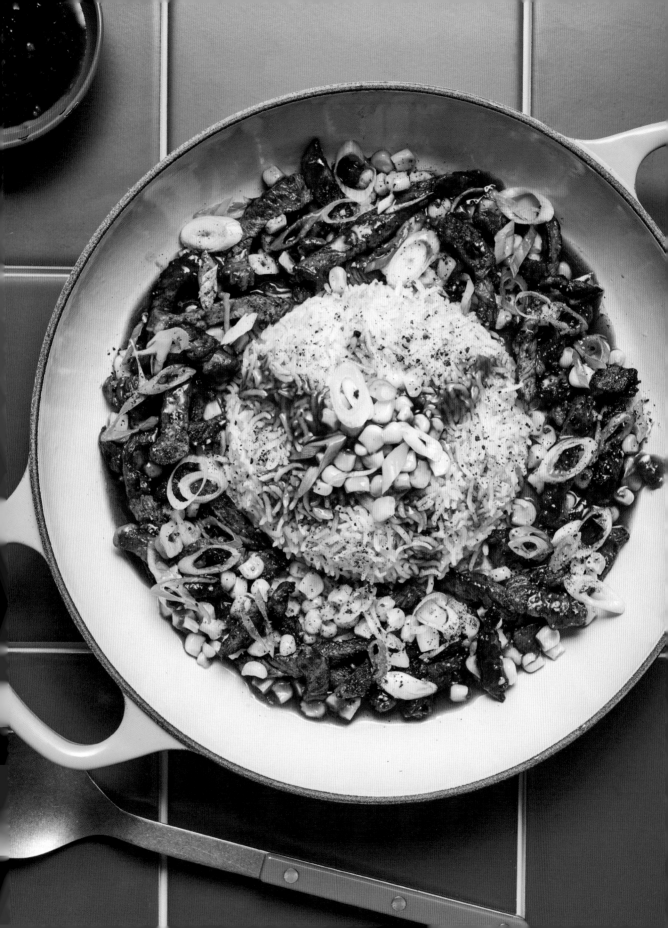

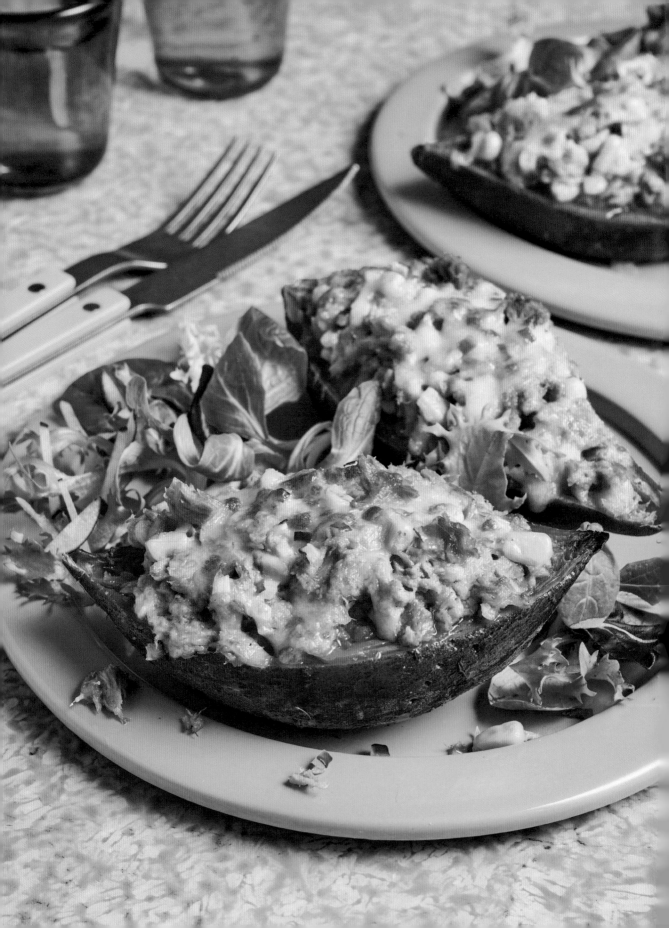

TUNA MELT LOADED SWEET POTATOES

SERVES: 2 | **PREP:** 2 MINS | **COOK:** 8–10 MINS

Tuna lovers, meet your ultimate loaded sweet potatoes. These may even convert the tuna haters. Tinned tuna makes a budget-friendly topping for a potato, with an extra melty finish, it's comforting and perfect for any night of the week.

2 medium sweet potatoes

3 slices of red onion, finely diced

4 tbsp tinned sweetcorn

224g drained tinned tuna in spring water

60g reduced-fat Cheddar, grated

60g reduced-fat mozzarella

½ tsp English mustard (optional)

1 tbsp mayonnaise (optional)

Salt and pepper

Side suggestion
Side salad

Swap: This works just as well with ordinary potatoes.

Pierce the sweet potatoes as many times as possible, then stick them in the microwave on high for 3 minutes on each side, but they may need longer depending on the size.

Meanwhile, mix all the remaining ingredients together. Once the sweet potatoes are cooked, slice them in half and then fluff up each centre.

Place the toppings on top and pop under a hot grill for a few minutes to melt the cheese.

Optional: Sometimes I like to mix in ½ teaspoon of any mustard and 1 tablespoon of mayonnaise to make it creamy!

Air fryer method: After piercing the potatoes, wrap them in foil and place in the air fryer at 200°C for 35–40 minutes or until cooked through.

KCAL	CARBS	PROTEIN	FAT		
378	39g	47g	5g		

HEARTY SAUSAGE CASSOULET WITH CROUTON TOPPING

SERVES: 4 | **PREP:** 5 MINS | **COOK:** 20–22 MINS | DF + NF

Cassoulet is traditionally a slow-cooked stew containing pork and white beans. But we're doing it the Very Hungry Greek way, so I've made mine much quicker, bursting with rosemary and thyme flavours. Mine comes complete with a homemade crouton topping to dip into the stewy goodness.

Low-calorie
  cooking spray
12 reduced-fat
  pork sausages
1 medium onion, diced
1 red pepper, diced
300g cherry tomatoes
2 garlic cloves, minced
400g tin chopped
  tomatoes
400g tin cannellini
  beans, drained
1 tsp dried thyme
1 tsp dried rosemary
100g vegetable stock
Salt and pepper

Croutons
90g wholemeal or
  white baguette,
  roughly torn
1 tbsp olive oil
1½ tsp paprika

Spray a large pan with low-calorie cooking spray and fry the sausages on a high heat for 3–4 minutes to get a nice colour on all sides. Remove from the pan and set aside.

Spray the same pan with more low-calorie cooking spray and fry the onion, red pepper, cherry tomatoes and garlic for 3–4 minutes. Then add the remaining ingredients and give them a good mix, then submerge the sausages under the other ingredients.

Simmer for 10 minutes, mixing halfway through and flattening the cherry tomatoes to release their juices.

To make the croutons, mix the torn bread with the olive oil and paprika, then scatter over the cassoulet. Place under a hot grill for a few minutes to brown. Serve and enjoy!

KCAL	CARBS	PROTEIN	FAT	
448	40g	30g	17g	

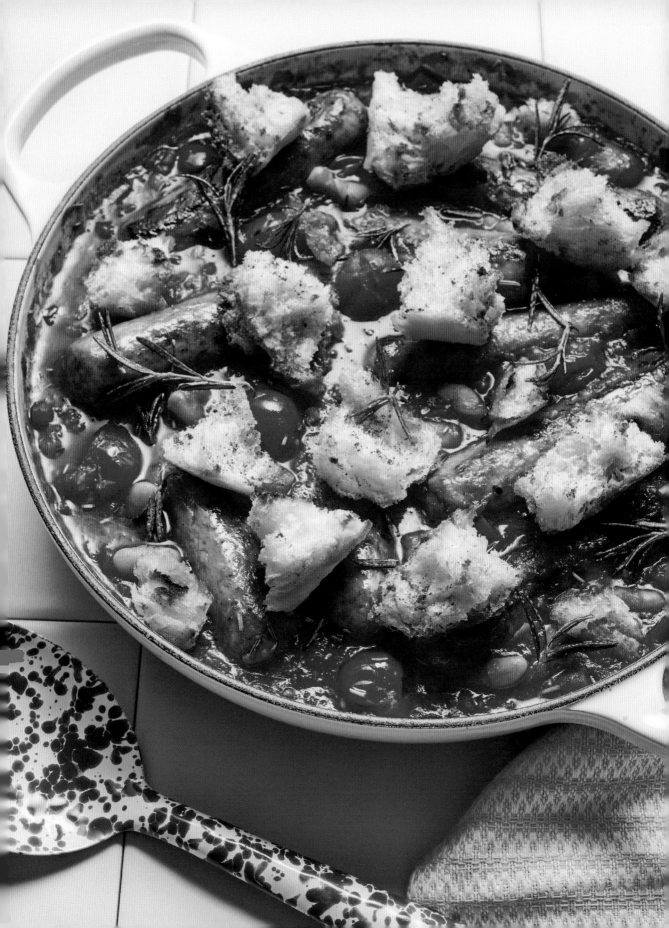

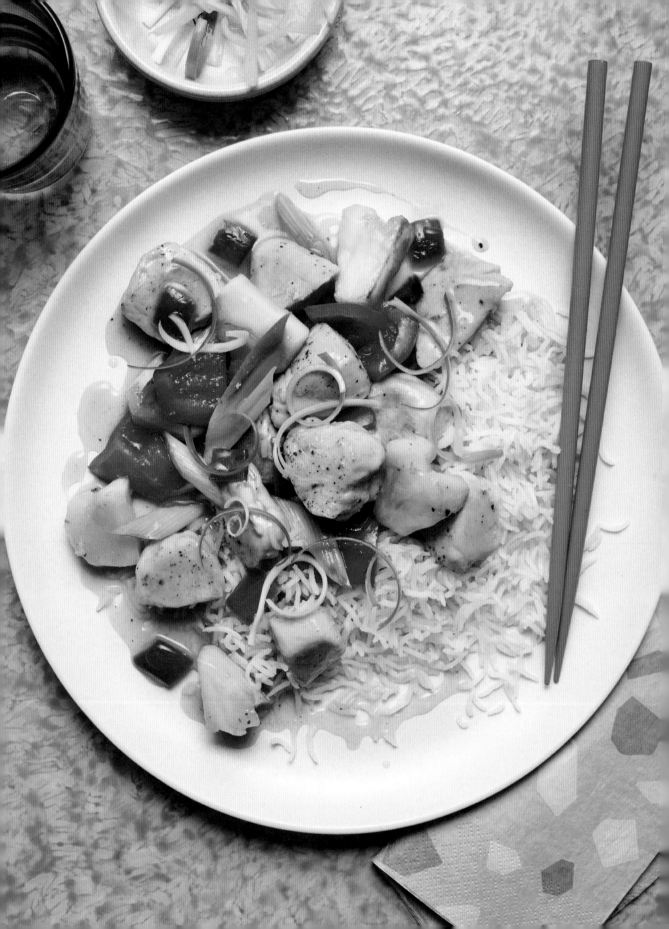

HAWAIIAN CHICKEN

SERVES: 4 | **PREP**: 5 MINS | **COOK**: 8–10 MINS | GF + DF + NF

The freshness of pineapple just sings in your mouth. So, if you're a pineapple lover like me and could eat it every day without getting sick of it, this Hawaiian chicken recipe will be right up your street!

4 chicken breasts, diced

Low-calorie cooking spray

2 red peppers

2 garlic cloves, minced

400g fresh pineapple, diced

2 spring onions, sliced

Salt and pepper

Sauce

200ml pineapple juice

1 tbsp soy sauce

½ chicken stockpot or cube

1 tsp cornflour, mixed with 2 tsp water

1 tsp sweetener (optional)

Side suggestion

Basmati rice

In a bowl, mix together all the sauce ingredients and set aside.

Season the chicken with a pinch of salt and pepper, then fry in a large frying pan sprayed with low-calorie cooking spray on a medium heat for 5–6 minutes until nearly cooked.

Add the peppers, garlic and pineapple and fry for a further 2 minutes, then crank up the heat to the highest temperature and add the sauce. Fry for 1–2 minutes or until the sauce reduces and everything is coated beautifully in the sauce. Sprinkle over the spring onions and enjoy!

Optional: Add a teaspoon of sweetener mixed in with the sauce (but taste it first!).

KCAL	CARBS	PROTEIN	FAT	
273	21g	42g	2g	

PARMESAN-CRUSTED CHICKEN AND BACON CAESAR SALAD

SERVES: 2 | **PREP:** 5 MINS | **COOK:** 8–10 MINS | GF + NF

With 69g of protein per serving, you'll be adding this twist on your standard Caesar salad to your weekly meal plan to reach your protein goals. The chicken is crusted with Parmesan and mixed with smoked bacon and delicious garlic croutons.

2 chicken breasts

40g Parmesan, grated

1 egg, beaten

Low-calorie cooking spray

50g gluten-free bread roll, cubed

1 garlic clove, minced

2 large handfuls of romaine lettuce

A handful of cherry tomatoes, sliced

4 cooked smoked bacon medallions, diced

2 soft-boiled eggs, halved

2 tbsp reduced-fat Caesar dressing

Salt and pepper

Butterfly each chicken breast, then cut all the way through so you've got two flat pieces per breast.

Grab a plate and mix the Parmesan together with a good pinch of black pepper. Dip each piece of chicken into the beaten egg, then the grated Parmesan mixture.

Spray a frying pan with plenty of low-calorie cooking spray and fry the chicken on a low–medium heat for 3 minutes on each side or until cooked. Remove from the pan and set aside.

In the same pan, spray the gluten-free croutons with low-calorie cooking spray, season with salt, pepper and the garlic. Fry for a few minutes to toast.

Slice the chicken, then assemble the salad on a plate along with the cooked bacon, homemade croutons and egg halves. Pour over the Caesar dressing and serve.

Air fryer method: Spray the chicken with low-calorie cooking spray and air-fry at 180°C for 8–10 minutes, flipping halfway.

KCAL	CARBS	PROTEIN	FAT	
488	15g	69g	17g	

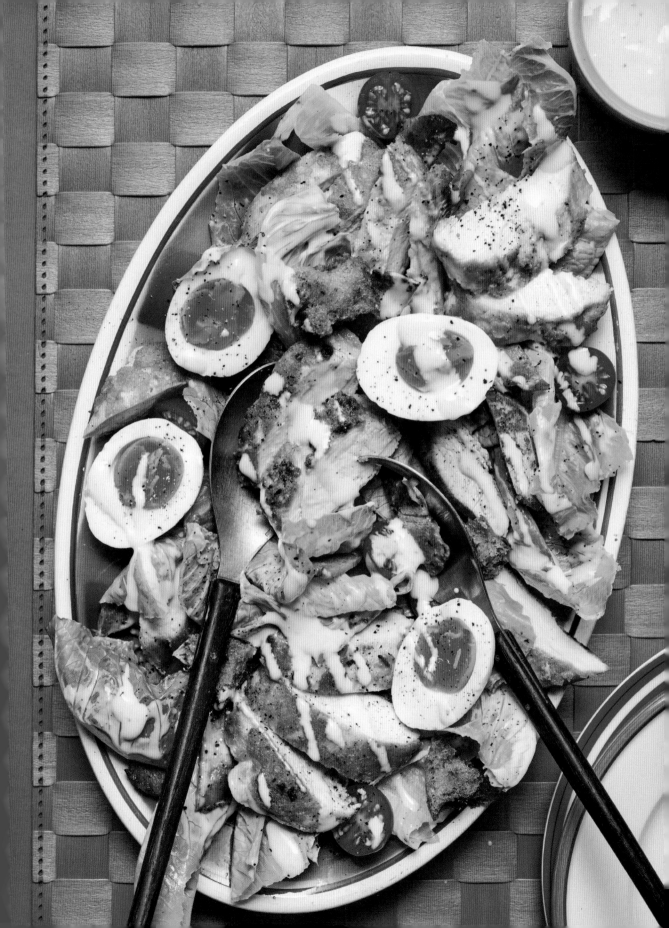

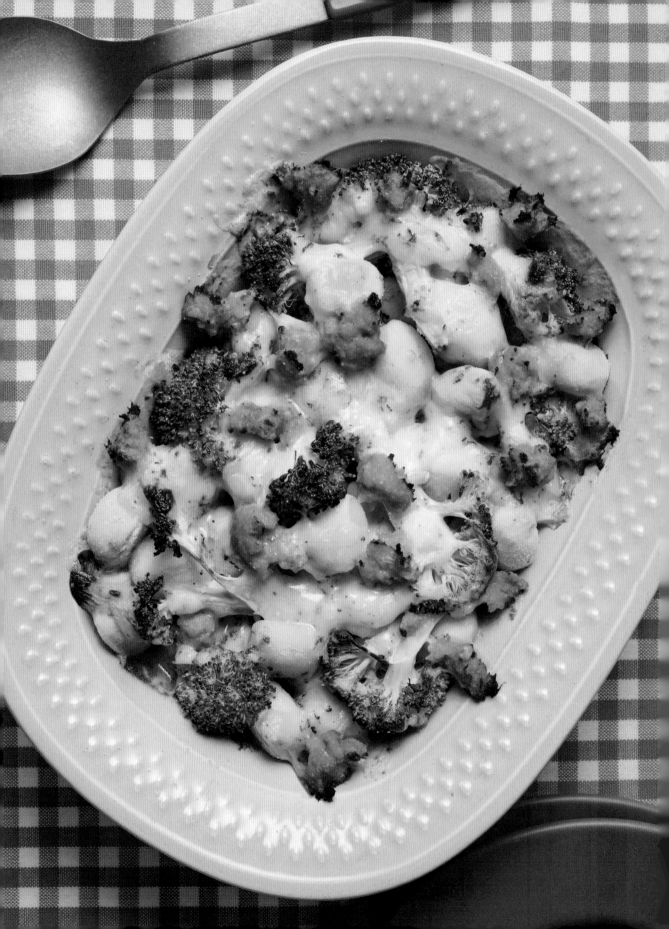

ROASTED BROCCOLI, SAUSAGE AND BLUE CHEESE GNOCCHI BAKE

SERVES: 2 | **PREP**: 5 MINS | **COOK**: 24–26 MINS | NF

I need to let you in on a little secret – I couldn't stand gnocchi when I was younger. How did I not like the fluffy, pillowy goodness of these little potato balls? Now, I cook with them every week without fail as they are so versatile and go with pretty much anything.

45g blue cheese, plus extra for topping if you like

100ml semi-skimmed milk

1 tsp cornflour mixed with 1 tbsp water to make a slurry

250g fresh gnocchi

130g broccoli, sliced

2 pork or vegetarian sausages, skin removed

Black pepper

Preheat the oven to 180°C.

Mix the blue cheese and semi-skimmed milk together in a pan on a low–medium heat until the cheese has melted, then mix in the cornflour slurry and cook on a low heat for 1–2 minutes until the sauce has thickened slightly.

Scatter the gnocchi and broccoli into a medium ovenproof dish and pour over the sauce. Break the sausages into small chunks over the top and add extra chunks of blue cheese if using.

Season with pepper and cook in the oven for 20 minutes.

Optional: Scatter over a few small chunks of blue cheese before baking and use veggie sausages to make this veggie.

Air fryer method: Air-fry at 200°C for 15–20 minutes.

KCAL	CARBS	PROTEIN	FAT
382	46g	19g	13g

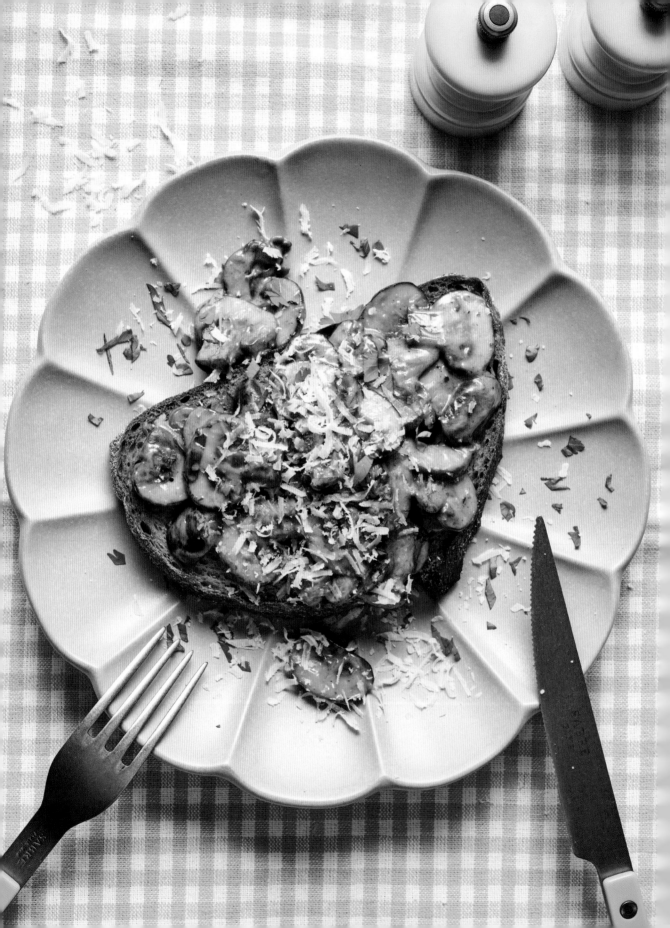

CREAMY MUSHROOMS ON TOAST

SERVES: 2 | **PREP**: 5 MINS | **COOK**: 4–6 MINS | V + NF

Am I the only person who can eat mushrooms raw? If you're a mushroom fan and you love a gourmet-tasting creamy sauce, give this a go.

Low-calorie cooking spray

300g chestnut mushrooms, sliced

1 garlic clove, minced

50g reduced-fat crème fraîche

2 slices of wholemeal sourdough, toasted

1–2 tbsp finely chopped fresh parsley

2 tbsp Parmesan, grated (optional)

Salt and pepper

Spray a frying pan with low-calorie cooking spray and fry the mushrooms with a pinch of salt and pepper for 3–4 minutes, then add the minced garlic.

Mix well and fry for a further 1–2 minutes, then stir in the crème fraîche. Top the toast with the mushrooms, sprinkle over the parsley and serve.

Optional: Scatter over some grated Parmesan with the parsley.

KCAL	CARBS	PROTEIN	FAT	
161	19g	7g	6g	

POLLO PESTO NAAN

SERVES: 2 | **PREP:** 5 MINS | **COOK:** 8–10 MINS | NF

If you need a quick lunch or dinner fix – look no further. It's a creamy pesto chicken dish on top of a yummy piece of naan. But you can also add this topping to whatever bread you fancy or mix it with pasta if you prefer.

2 chicken breasts, sliced

Low-calorie cooking spray

8 mushrooms, sliced

¼ red onion, sliced

40g light soft cheese

1 tbsp reduced-fat green pesto

2 mini naans

30g reduced-fat mozzarella

Salt and pepper

Side suggestion

A handful of watercress

Season the sliced chicken with salt and pepper. Spray a pan with low-calorie cooking spray and cook the chicken for 3–4 minutes, then add the mushrooms and red onion.

Fry for a further 3–4 minutes, then mix in the soft cheese, pesto and a splash of water. Pop the naans in the toaster, then load them up with the chicken mixture and tear over the mozzarella.

Stick the naans under a hot grill to melt the cheese and serve.

KCAL	CARBS	PROTEIN	FAT
430	34g	50g	9g

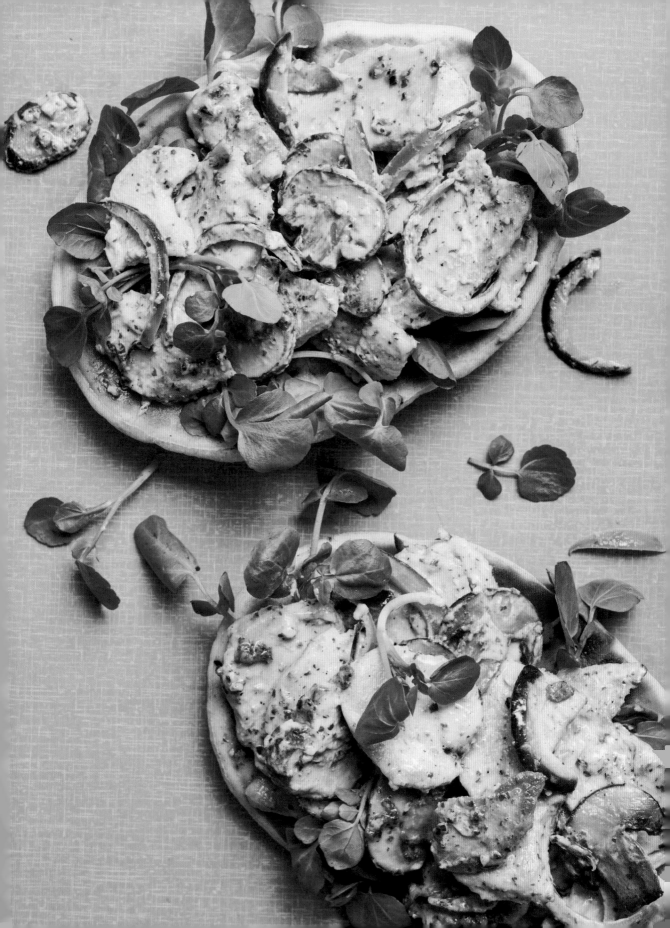

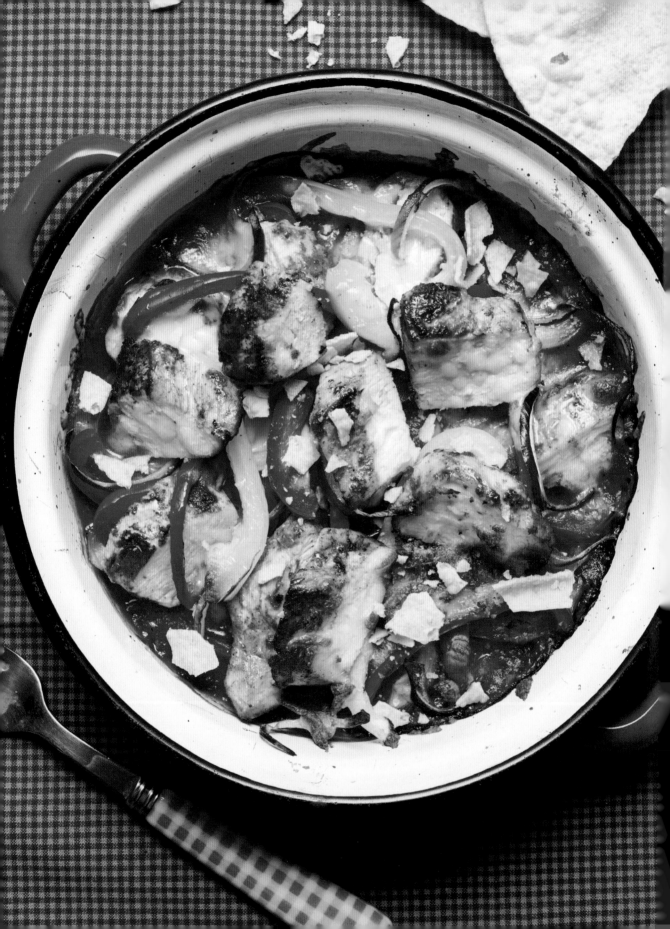

TANDOORI CHICKEN BOWLS

SERVES: 2 | **PREP**: 5 MINS | **COOK**: 23–28 MINS | GF + NF

These tandoori chicken bowls are crammed full of flavours and fillings. But don't forget the side suggestions to take them to the next level!

2 chicken breasts

Low-calorie cooking spray

100g passata

1 tbsp tomato purée

1 tsp garam masala

Pinch of salt

60g reduced-fat mozzarella, torn or grated

¼ red onion, sliced

½ red pepper, sliced

½ yellow pepper, sliced

Tandoori marinade

1 tbsp tandoori seasoning

2 heaped tbsp fat-free Greek yogurt

2.5cm piece of fresh ginger, peeled and minced

2 garlic cloves, minced

Juice of ½ lemon

1 tbsp tomato purée

Side suggestions

Mint sauce and ½ poppadom per person, crushed, over each bowl for a texture sensation

Butterfly the chicken breasts, then slice all the way through, so you've got two flat pieces per breast. Mix all the tandoori marinade ingredients together in a bowl, then add the chicken and leave to marinate for at least 30 minutes.

Preheat the oven to 180°C.

Spray a frying pan with low-calorie cooking spray and fry the marinated chicken on a medium heat for 4 minutes on each side. Leave it to rest, then slice.

Mix the passata, tomato purée, garam masala and salt together, then spread over the bottom of two small ovenproof dishes. In layers, add half the cheese, a layer of the veg, the chicken, more veg then the rest of the cheese.

Cook in the oven for 15 minutes.

Optional: Add a dash of red food colouring to the marinade for a vibrant tandoori colour.

Air fryer method: Air-fry the ovenproof dishes at 180°C for 12–14 minutes.

KCAL	CARBS	PROTEIN	FAT
331	14g	54g	6g

INDEX

ABOUT THE AUTHOR

Christina Kynigos is a super enthusiastic, Greek-Cypriot foodie who doesn't do things by halves or stick to the rules. Going above and beyond, Christina has created these healthy recipes to push the boat out on what's achievable in low-calorie cooking, changing the healthy food game forever.

She got her name from having a super healthy appetite and her ethnicity. There's nothing in the world that gives her more joy than seeing people eat and enjoy the food she cooks. That doesn't mean just Greek food either; Christina experiments with cuisines from all around the world, expanding her palate and inspiring others to do the same.

Christina started the Very Hungry Greek in 2020 and now has a following of over 240k around the world on both Instagram and TikTok. This is her second cookbook.

ACKNOWLEDGEMENTS

This second book wouldn't have been possible without the support of all my social media followers. You loved the first book so much that it was possible to produce a second book and for that, I owe you everything.

Thank you to my family, especially my grandparents, who brought me up around food and ignited my passion for cooking. My yiayia and bapou (grandma and grandad) said to always follow my dreams and supported me along every single path in life.

Thank you to my dear friends who are my cheerleaders. You always egg me on and give me confidence to banish my self-doubt; you're the best.

And lastly thank you to YOU, the reader, for buying my book and wanting to try my recipes.

You are all truly incredible.

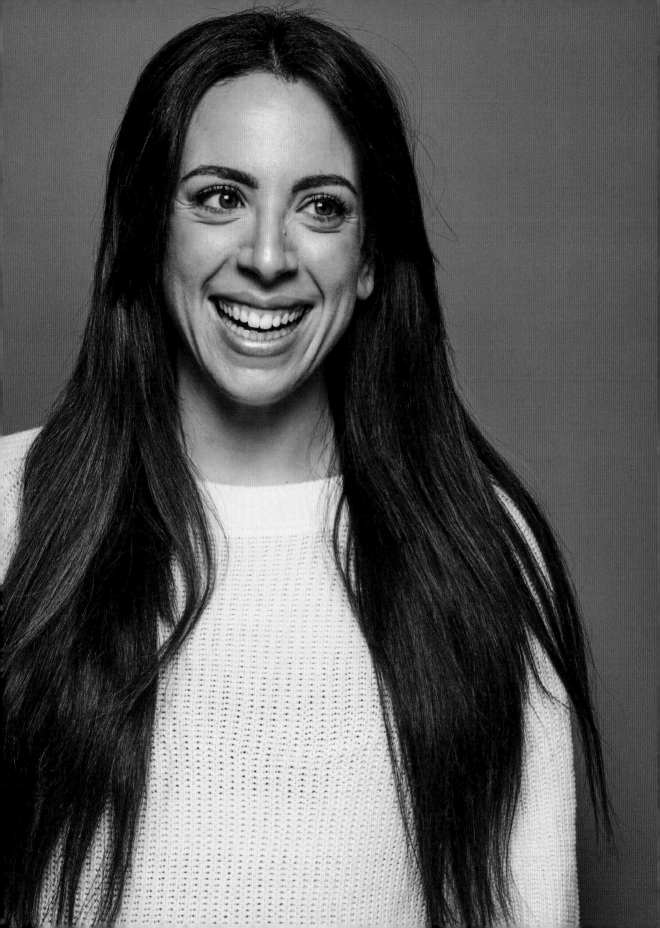

METRIC/IMPERIAL CONVERSION CHART

All equivalents are rounded, for practical convenience.

WEIGHT	
25g	1oz
50g	2oz
100g	3½oz
150g	5oz
200g	7oz
250g	9oz
300g	10oz
400g	14oz
500g	1lb 2oz
1 kg	2¼lb

VOLUME (LIQUIDS)		
5ml		1 tsp
15ml		1 tbsp
30ml	1fl oz	⅛ cup
60ml	2fl oz	¼ cup
75ml		⅓ cup
120ml	4fl oz	½ cup
150ml	5fl oz	⅔ cup
175ml		¾ cup
250ml	8fl oz	1 cup
1 litre	1 quart	4 cups

OVEN TEMPERATURES		
Fan	°C	°F
120	140	275
130	150	300
140	160	325
160	180	350
170	190	375
180	200	400
200	220	425
210	230	450

LENGTH	
1cm	½ inch
2.5cm	1 inch
20cm	8 inches
25cm	10 inches
30cm	12 inches

VOLUME (DRY INGREDIENTS – AN APPROXIMATE GUIDE)	
butter	1 cup (2 sticks) = 225g
rolled oats	1 cup = 100g
fine powders (e.g. flour)	1 cup = 125g
breadcrumbs (fresh)	1 cup = 50g
breadcrumbs (dried)	1 cup = 125g
nuts (e.g. almonds)	1 cup = 125g
seeds (e.g. chia)	1 cup = 160g
dried fruit (e.g. raisins)	1 cup = 150g
dried legumes (large, e.g. chickpeas)	1 cup = 170g
grains, granular goods and small dried legumes (e.g. rice, quinoa, sugar, lentils)	1 cup = 200g
grated cheese	1 cup = 100g